Solutions
FOR
Adults
WITH
ASPERGER SYNDROME

Solutions
FOR
Adults
WITH
ASPERGER
SYNDROME

Maximizing the Benefits, Minimizing the Drawbacks to Achieve Success

JUANITA P. LOVETT, PH.D.

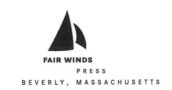

FAIR WINDS
PRESS
BEVERLY, MASSACHUSETTS

First published in the USA in 2005 by
Fair Winds Press, a member of
Quayside Publishing Group
100 Cummings Center
Suite 406-L
Beverly, MA 01915-6101
www.fairwindspress.com

09 08   3 4 5

ISBN-13: 978-1-059233-164-2
ISBN-10: 1-59233-164-5

Library of Congress Cataloging-in-Publication Data available

Book design by *tabula rasa* graphic design

*The information in this book is for educational purposes only. It is
not intended to replace the advice of a physician or medical practi-
tioner. Please see your health care provider before beginning any new
health program.*

To my daughter, Laura, whose help made it happen.
To Terry T., who first named Asperger's syndrome for me.
And to the families who helped me to understand AS.

Contents

PART II: LIVING WITH AS

"Psychologist Juanita Lovett drew on her years of experience working with adults with Asperger Syndrome (AS) to create a book that clearly and accurately describes AS, its characteristics, and how it presents itself in adulthood. In addition to providing valuable and much needed resources, she uses real-life examples to explain the impact of the diagnosis on adults, their relationships, and those who love and work with them. This book is a welcome and valuable resource, and I will happily recommend it to OASIS visitors."

—Barbara Kirby, co-author of *The OASIS Guide to Asperger Syndrome* and founder of the OASIS (Online Asperger Syndrome Information and Support) Web site at www.aspergersyndrome.org.

Foreword

This book encompasses the once overlooked needs of adults with AS and also the needs of the families who love and care for them. Dr. Jaunita P. Lovett, Ph.D. explains some of the classic AS behaviors that until now have been hidden from medical professionals and other segments of society—behaviors often labeled "family secrets" and kept behind closed doors by families living with AS.

The American Psychiatric Association did not recognize AS in its *Diagnostic and Statistical Manual of Mental Disorders: Fourth Edition,* or DSM-IV, until 1994 in the U.S., and then it was only in children. But children have a way of growing into adulthood; and children who have AS will also have the disorder as adults. For some unknown reason, medical professionals in the past ignored this fact and because of their miscalculations adults with AS have been completely ignored.

Adults who have AS are found throughout all segments of society—in every corner of every country in the world.

Society has benefited from individuals suspected of having AS—including such great minds as Van Gogh, Einstein, and Bach. Of course, because they are no longer living, these talented geniuses cannot be officially diagnosed, but their personal stories are part of history. Geniuses with AS have opened our hearts and our eyes to beautiful art and music and our minds to new frontiers of thought.

Thanks to Dr. Lovett's book and the efforts of many other professionals and nonprofessionals alike, society is becoming more informed about autistic spectrum disorders and, more specifically, AS in adults and how it affects other family members.

More understanding and services are needed for assistance and support for adults with AS and their families. Only then will millions of people be given a chance to realize and cope with the reality that individuals with AS may think and act differently. These individuals are not "broken" or "bad." They don't need to be "fixed." They are simply different.

The stigma of autism spectrum disorders will begin to diminish as soon as truthful information is offered to the public regarding these neurological/biological disorders and they are understood and accepted as part of the human condition.

Solutions for Adults with Asperger Syndrome is a book I highly recommend to adults with AS, their families, professionals, educators, and anyone who works with the public. AS is all around us. Your life and your ability to better understand AS could benefit greatly by reading this book.

Ignorance breeds intolerance, and intolerance is unacceptable.

Karen E. Rodman,
Director and Founder, Families of Adults Afflicted with Asperger's Syndrome (FAAAS), Inc., http://www.faaas.org

Introduction

"For so long, the idea that Asperger Syndrome [AS] occurs in adults has been so taboo that by reading the textbooks on AS, one would be left with the impression that AS is miraculously cured or is uniformly fatal at age 18."

This quote is from a health care professional who has personally experienced the impact of Asperger Syndrome (AS). After having one child diagnosed as autistic and a second diagnosed as having AS, she realized that her husband shared many of the same characteristics, such as problems with communication and difficulties with understanding relationships. These characteristics had caused many problems in their marriage, but her husband refused to be evaluated. This prompted his wife to begin searching for information in the medical literature about AS in adults, hoping to better understand her husband and to improve their relationship. To her frustration, she found little helpful information. Although there was information about AS in children, there was very little research looking at AS in adults to help her understand the syndrome.

Becoming Aware of AS

When I first became aware of AS as a new diagnostic category, I was struck by how well the pattern of symptoms matched characteristics of some individuals that I had seen as patients over my twenty-five years of practice as a clinical psychologist. I had also encountered these characteristics in a number of people I had come across in my "organizational effectiveness" consulting work for large, high-tech organizations. These patients and employees had never really fit any of the existing diagnostic categories because of their unusual pattern of symptoms and abilities. Many of these people were brilliant, and some were professionally quite successful. But all of them had difficulty with intimate relationships and were uncomfortable dealing with social situations. Some had special interests, often unusual, that preoccupied them, sometimes to the point of dominating their lives. Many had "scripts" that they routinely used to deal with other people. Their difficulties began when the scripts weren't enough—when the relationship demanded more than just formalities. In these cases, it quickly became clear that these individuals struggled with understanding interpersonal relationships despite their very high IQs. The suburban location where I practiced contained many exceptionally gifted patients, yet these extremely intelligent people seemed unable to grasp the role they had played in the problems they had with other people. AS as a diagnosis seemed to offer the explanation for their problems. I decided that I needed to learn more about AS, and I began to look for sources of professional education such as professional conferences and publications that would tell me more about this syndrome. At that time, the only available information focused on children. Like the health care professional quoted above, I was frustrated that there was almost no information on AS in adults.

AS Is a Mystifying Syndrome

AS is a syndrome that seems to mystify the people who become involved with it. Many people with AS are very intelligent and often have unusual abilities, such as a remarkable memory for facts or an uncanny ability to solve mathematical calculations. These abilities often coexist with difficulties in communication, an inability to understand other people's perspectives, problems with social interactions, and a tendency to be obsessed with a special interest in some unusual area (for example, trains and railroad timetables or complex mathematical equations). It is difficult to make sense of this unusual pattern of strengths and weaknesses, and this is what mystifies people. The question that is so compelling is this: "How is it possible for someone to be so exceptional in understanding some things and yet seem to have little or no ability to understand other kinds of things, especially ones that involve other people?"

The syndrome can also be very puzzling to people who have AS. In many cases, these individuals realize that they are different and that it is hard for them to fit in or be accepted by others. But the very nature of the syndrome (which is what the first part of this book is about) interferes with the person's ability to understand his or her differences. These differences in thinking and understanding interfere with the ability to have satisfactory interpersonal relationships or sometimes even have their career of choice. The condition is also troubling to the people around individuals with AS because they can't figure out what causes so much miscommunication between them and the person with AS.

The Purpose of the Book

This book is intended to help individuals diagnosed with AS, and the people who live with them, to learn about AS. Learning about AS and gaining an understanding of how AS affects who has it will make clearer, in turn, how AS affects the individual the people who are a part of his or her life. The book is based on what I have learned about AS from many sources. The sources include my work with individuals who have the diagnosis of AS and who have generously shared their stories. I've included information from people who, after reading about AS, have self-diagnosed. There will be information from spouses and families of people with AS that will help make clear how AS affects the lives of individuals who live with AS in their midst. I've included information about what researchers are learning about this still not understood condition, as well as some of the theories that have been generated to try to explain the unusual pattern of abilities and differences in the way people with AS think and function. And, finally, I've included information and understanding that I've gained from colleagues who also work with individuals with AS. My goal is to put this information together in a way that will be helpful to individuals who are just becoming aware of AS and need to both understand it and find practical solutions to dealing with the differences in the way people with AS approach the world.

How This Book Is Organized

The book is organized in two parts, reflecting the approach that I have found most helpful in dealing with my patients who have AS or individuals who have someone with AS in their life. Part I,

Learning About AS, is designed to help the reader gain an understanding of what the syndrome is, why it has been difficult for many adults to get the correct diagnosis, and the important theories about the nature of the syndrome. The last chapter of Part I looks at the key research findings about the differences in the structure and function of the AS brain compared with the brains of people who do not have AS and how these finding may help to explain the syndrome.

The intent of Part II, Living with AS, is to provide an understanding of how having AS affects the life of the person with AS as well as the people around him or her. Throughout the book, I've provided a number of examples of how AS affects the individual's behavior and of AS-NT interactions. I've found in my work that these "verbal pictures" are essential to understanding the impact of AS. The examples will illustrate some of the strategies used by people with AS to cope with their lives as well as the problems they face in dealing with a world that can be very confusing. The examples will also show how AS behavior can often baffle and frustrate the people around the person with AS. I believe, and my work with patients confirms, that the most effective way to help people with AS and their families is to help them understand how AS affects their lives and to recognize those incidents when AS is playing a role in problems or misunderstandings that occur. By understanding AS, it is possible to identify some practical solutions to dealing with it.

Notes About This Book
The examples used throughout this book are taken from real life, but I have altered identifying information and changed circumstances to assure anonymity. I am very grateful to the people

who, by telling me about their lives and supporting the writing of this book, are helping to reach out to build a bridge between individuals with AS and the rest of the people with whom they share this world.

Two other points: I have used "we" in writing much of this book because so much of what I know and I have written about is the result of a great deal of consultation with others knowledgeable about AS (including patients) and their willingness to share their knowledge. It's important to me to acknowledge that what is written here is the result of the effort on the part of many to help make AS understandable. The second point concerns gender usage. Rather than to always use the awkward he or she, him or her, himself or herself, and so on, I've chosen to rely primarily on "he" and "him." I made this decision because the majority of people I have worked with who have AS are male, and, currently, there are more males being diagnosed with AS than females, although I believe that is more an artifact of the diagnostic criteria than the truth. The diagnostic criteria will likely be revised as we know more about AS, but at present, the ratio of males to females being diagnosed with AS is 4:1.

Finally, this book is not intended as a professional text on AS nor does it attempt to cover every aspect of AS. Instead, it is written, based on the patients and families that I saw or information I learned from professional colleagues, with the goal of being helpful to people with AS and their families and significant others. I hoped to write what I wished so many times I could have found—an introduction and overview of AS and some practical solutions for dealing with it.

CHAPTER ONE

Understanding Asperger Syndrome and Its History

Diana walked quietly into the office. It was obvious that she had been crying. Her face looked tired and drawn under her Florida tan, and her skirt hung loosely around her waist. She had told me at our first meeting that she was having trouble sleeping and had lost her appetite. She chose a straight-backed chair and sat with her hands clasped in her lap. Tom walked in a few steps behind her, his posture and pace strangely like hers except for his lack of arm movement. He too took a straight-backed chair, and curiously he reached out and took her hand. I knew that he had asked Diana for a divorce to "see if he could be happy" with a woman he had met—a clerk in the organization where he was a senior manager. Neither of them spoke.

I asked them how the past week had been. Diana had asked him to come to couples' counseling to see if they could save their marriage. This had been several weeks ago. Although Tom had come willingly, he had stated during the first meeting that he knew that once he had decided to do something, he had to go ahead, whether it was right or wrong. I'd noticed that he was able to cite examples of things Diana had done that he saw as wrong, but he took no responsibility for causing marital difficulties himself. In fact, he became upset if Diana tried to tell her side of the story or to talk about the things Tom had done that were hurtful. I wondered if that was why Diana wasn't talking.

Tom looked out the window and then said, "I wish we could hurry this up. I want to get this over with." I saw tears sliding down Diana's cheeks. She looked at him and looked away. Last week, he was telling me how "mean" Diana was to him and that all he wanted was a chance to be happy. I had asked him for an example of how she was mean. He said she got upset and angry and complained about the work she had to do to prepare for family visits. I knew he came from a large extended family and wondered about the demands of living in a big house on the beach, which his family seemed to view as a vacation hotel.

Tom began talking about some detective novel he had just read. He said, "At the end of the book, the detective and the woman he had saved decided to buy a house in Key West to spend the rest of their lives together. That's what I want." He turned and announced to Diana, "I just want to be happy." He looked at her again and said, "You won't have any trouble finding someone to be with. You're very pretty, and some people seem to like you. The only problem you will have is figuring out whether men want you or your money. With the divorce settlement, you'll be rich." My heart dropped. No matter how often I hear the blunt language of Asperger Syndrome, it still has an impact on me.

Diana's shoulders shook while she held in sobs. Tom was annoyed. "Why are you crying again?"

I knew that Diana was having trouble handling Tom's comments. She was still in shock from finding out that the man she loved and believed loved her had been having an affair for the last three years with a woman who was twenty years younger than he was. During that time, Tom admitted he had never told her that he was upset or unhappy. He simply said, "She should have known." How she should have known was never made clear.

During the three years that he was having the affair, he had put pressure on Diana to leave her profession and move to the home in Florida he had insisted they buy. It was clear to me Tom had no idea what he had done to his wife, moving her from her hometown, where she had many friends and a support network, to a new place, while at the same time planning to leave her and get a divorce. From his perspective, he had found someone new who was very impressed with him, and he wanted to try that relationship to see if he would be happy. He insisted that Diana wasn't a bad person, but he had decided to get a divorce, and he had to go ahead with it. Diana had told me when I first saw her that Tom's original proposal was that he would like to take turns, living with her first and then the other woman for two-month periods. That way he could tell which one made him happier.

His AS logic was devastating to his wife. Tom had no interest in looking at himself and, in fact, took the position that he was who he was. Diana would need to pick up the pieces of her life and move on.

Tom has Asperger Syndrome (AS). He has been quite successful at the technology company where he works, but he has trouble understanding interpersonal issues or seeing another person's perspective. These "blind spots" are a result of his AS. Tom is very smart. Over the years, he has learned how to compensate for some of the differences in the way he thinks, but under stressful or emotionally charged conditions, his coping skills often fail, and his actions and words can be insensitive and hurtful. He is more focused on the present than on the future and doesn't always anticipate the consequences of his behavior, especially if it requires him to understand another person's state of mind. AS can be a confusing, frustrating condition, and we are just beginning to gain some understanding of the syndrome in adults and what it means to both those who have it and those around them.

Misunderstandings About Asperger Syndrome

There is a common misunderstanding that AS is a mental illness. This is not the case. AS is a neurodevelopmental condition that is at the most able end of a group of developmental disorders. Neurodevelopmental refers to the development and growth of neurons, the cells that make up the tissue of the brain. In the case of AS, this growth does not follow the usual progression of development. The result is a brain that processes information differently than that of most people. This group of developmental disorders is referred to as the "pervasive developmental disorders" (PDDs) because they affect so many areas of the individual's life throughout the lifespan. AS, like the rest of the PDDs, is a developmental difference, not a delay, in the way some areas of the brain function (see Chapter Five for more on AS and the brain). It results in certain differences in the way the brain processes information, especially that of a social nature. It is neither outgrown nor curable. While there is not full agreement at this time, most experts view AS as a mild variant of autism.

Myths About AS
• AS is a mental illness.
• AS is a children's disorder.
• AS can be cured with medication.
• AS will be outgrown.
• Faulty parenting causes AS.

Truths About AS
• AS is not a mental illness; it is a neurobiological difference.
• AS is a lifelong condition.
• AS is hardwired; at present, there is no medication for it.
• AS will not be outgrown, although the person may develop ways to cope with it.
• The cause of AS is not fully understood, but genetics play a major role.

What Is AS and Autism?

The autism spectrum disorders have three major characteristics in common: difficulty with communication, difficulty with social relationships, and the inability to understand another's state of mind. This triad is thought to be the result of a series of inefficiencies in brain functioning related to the structures and pathways that allow neurotypical (NT) individuals to register and process multiple channels of input at the same time. Autism and AS share these same fundamental problems and, for that reason, they are thought to be variants of the same disorder that differ in degree of severity.

Other Characteristics of AS
IQ and Verbal Issues

Individuals with AS have higher IQs than individuals in the rest of the autism spectrum, ranging from normal to very superior.

ℜ

AS OR AUTISM?

AS and autism share some key characteristics, but in order for the diagnosis of AS to be made, the individual must have a relatively normal intelligence level and no history of delay in the development of language.

⤬

THE AUTISTIC TRIAD

• Difficulty with communication
• Difficulty with social relationships
• Inability to understand others' state of mind

The diagnostic criteria included in the Diagnostic and Statistical Manual of Mental Disorders: Fourth Edition (DSM-IV-R) of the American Psychiatric Association state that in order to diagnose AS rather than autism, the individual must meet the normal milestones for speech development. Frequently, however, they do have verbal differences, such as speaking in a monotone voice, using an unusually loud or soft voice, and using words in a literal way.

Julie walked into my office and slumped into a chair. "I feel sometimes like I am crazy...even now when Jack has been diagnosed with AS. I still feel as if I've stepped through the looking glass." I asked her to give me an example of what makes her feel "crazy," so we could talk about it. "Like last night, Jack's mother was visiting us. I asked Jack to see if she would like some tea. He went upstairs, and I went to put the kettle on. I made the tea, and since Jack hadn't said his mother wanted any, I put two cups on the tray for him and me. He asked, 'Where is Mom's cup?' I said, did you ask her if she wants some? He answered, 'Of course, and she does want some.' I was frustrated that he had asked her but didn't bother to tell me her answer. I asked, "Why didn't you tell me?" He responded, 'You didn't tell me to tell you. You just said to ask her, and I did.'" This is an example of how individuals with AS can baffle others when they use language in a completely literal way.

Many clinicians with extensive experience working with AS question the diagnostic requirement that the AS child must have normal verbal development. Careful examination of many children who have the other symptoms of AS (the triad of difficulty with communication, with social relating, and with understanding the minds of others) reveals that in many cases, there were differences in verbal development. The DSM-IV-R is currently being revised, and the revision may reflect some of this thinking.

Special Interests

Individuals with AS often have special interests that may be repetitive and quite restrictive. Such special interests often include a fascination with facts and numbers, such as dates and telephone numbers, or a particular interest in things that involve mobility, such as trains, railroad timetables, highway maps, routes, and distances. While these interests may change over time, the obsessiveness of the interest remains unchanged.

A young college student with AS who had a longstanding interest in sports statistics became concerned with the fact that stadiums all over the country were changing their names as the result of commercial contracts. He began studying the changes, reporting on them to everyone he met, and writing letters to officials saying that he thought this was wrong. He spent endless amounts of time on the Internet trying to find out what stadium might be the next to make such a change. His pursuit of this became so intense that, although an honor student, his grades began to suffer.

Motor Coordination

There are other characteristics frequently seen in AS, such as a lack of motor coordination that may range from subtle to quite noticeable. A frequently seen example of this is a rather unusual walk that includes a deficient synchronization of leg and arm movement. People with AS are often clumsy and can have difficulty with knowing where their body is in space. As a result, they may stand too close to others or bump into objects.

When I first began studying this syndrome, I remember my surprise when an experienced colleague noted a patient leaving the clinic and advised me to note his walk. The client's arms remained at his side, unmoving as he walked out of the office. She described it as a sign of AS. A later case conference confirmed the diagnosis. I've since noted this lack of synchronization in my own work with adults with AS. It tends to be especially noticeable when the person is stressed or overtired.

NT—NEUROTYPICAL

The term used to characterize individuals who do not have AS is "neurotypical," or NT, which we will use in this book to refer to non-AS individuals.

Resistance to Change

Most people with AS have difficulty with change—they have a very powerful need for sameness and predictability. One patient described that she feels safe when things are predictable. Others describe the very real discomfort they experience when routines are disturbed. These changes in routine frequently result in behaviors that are attempts to control the situation to avoid discomfort. NTs often interpret these behaviors as selfish, callous, or uncaring. Those with AS also resist change in their environment and become upset if, for example, the furniture in a room is rearranged.

A man whose wife has AS described a very painful memory of being suddenly struck by severe chest pain as they prepared to take their weekly trip to the local airport where they were going to pick up his teenage stepchildren. His wife's response was to tell him that it was time to go to the airport; he could come or not as he pleased. He told her he was afraid he was having a heart attack, and she responded, "Call 911."

Inflexibility

People with AS have trouble being flexible. They do not like changes in their routine or their environment. AS thinking is also inflexible. Once people with AS make a decision, it is difficult or impossible to get them to change their mind. It is also very difficult for someone with the syndrome to look at something in a different way or even to shift his or her attention to something else.

A college student reported that he had to skip class and go home when the person with whom he rode took a different route to school. He explained that it was because he couldn't "settle down and study." He went on to say that he needed things to go in the right order to be able to move on to the next thing and be able to concentrate.

Behaviors like this create a great deal of frustration for people around individuals with AS. Others do not always understand that the action reflects the differences in how the AS brain functions.

One spouse reported feeling furious with her husband (who has AS) when he refused to eat any food that had come in contact with any other food on his plate. He would become quite upset and demand a clean plate and fresh food.

Response to Stimuli

Individuals with AS often have unusual responses to stimuli. Adults with AS may either over- or under-respond to heat, cold, or pain. They may be unable to tolerate certain sounds such as the whine of a hair dryer or the sound of a kitchen fan. Sensitivities may even extend to certain colors. It is hard for NTs to understand these sensory problems, but one way they could relate to these sensitivities is to think about how most people respond to nails scratching on a blackboard.

The mother of a young-adult son with AS reported that he could not stand for anything green to be in a meal served to him. Her son commented that green made him feel nauseated. Also, he could not stand the sound of the kitchen exhaust fan. To him, it sounded like a jet engine inside his head.

Summary of AS Symptoms
• Difficulty with communication
• Difficulty with social relationships
• Inability to understand others' state of mind
• Verbal differences (too loud/too soft voice, literal use of language)
• Intense special interests
• Problems with motor coordination
• Difficulty with change
• Inflexible routines
• Unusual response to stimuli

The Impact of AS
Within the AS diagnosis, there is a wide range in the degree to which a given individual is affected. Some individuals seem to

be only mildly affected, while others are not able to manage their daily life. But in all cases, the impact of AS on the way the person with AS thinks, acts, and reacts to others often causes pain, confusion, and frustration for all concerned. From these examples, which are multiplied many times a day in different forms, it is clear that although AS is at the higher-functioning end of the autism spectrum, it is a serious condition that needs to be identified.

Getting a Diagnosis

The symptoms of AS involve many areas of thinking and behaving. The exact form that these symptoms take may look somewhat different because of the unique personality of the individual. I have worked with adults with AS who love to brew beer, do yoga, and run big businesses; are shy or love to be the center of attention. As a result, I am often reminded that, "If you've seen one Aspie, you've seen one Aspie!" We are all born with certain personality traits, such as shy, talkative, and so on. As we grow up, our environment affects us, and that coupled with our personality traits makes us the people we are. The fact that AS is a difference in the way the brain works has a powerful impact on who the AS individual becomes, but AS is only one aspect of who the person is. Adults with AS demonstrate the same variability we all do. These differences mean that it is important for the clinician to be very familiar with the syndrome in order to recognize it as it presents itself in that person.

If a diagnosis of AS is suspected, it is best to consult with clinicians or centers that are familiar with the autism spectrum. This will require some research, but a misdiagnosis or being told there is no diagnosis could have serious implications with regard to accessing the right treatment and needed services. It may mean that the person and his or her significant others are denied the opportunity to find solutions to dealing with AS.

Individuals with a great deal of experience with the syndrome find AS easy to recognize, because the fundamental similarities can be detected with the right questioning. And when the clinician has input from not just the adult with AS but from others who know the adult with AS well, verification of the diagnosis becomes quite straightforward.

Why is it difficult to find someone who is able to diagnose AS?
One factor that contributes to the problem of getting an accurate assessment is that AS is a relatively new diagnosis in the United States. The American Psychiatric Association's DSM-IV-R,

the source of diagnostic codes for mental health professionals in the United States, did not include the diagnosis of AS until its 1994 edition. There have been several revisions to the criteria for the diagnosis, and there is still a lack of broad consensus as to what symptoms should make up the diagnosis and how severe they must be to be officially recognized. Further complicating the picture is that not all people with AS will exhibit all the behaviors listed in the DSM-IV-R.

A History of the Diagnosis of AS
Kanner's Autism

AS as a diagnosis has only been recognized in the United States since 1994. Before that, autism disorder in the U.S. was defined by the work of Dr. Leo Kanner. In 1943, Dr. Kanner identified a type of disorder where a child, more often a boy, demonstrated a set of behaviors that included severe withdrawal from the world, social indifference manifested as a lack of interest in others (a pervasive remoteness), language difficulties, narrow interests, and repetitive behaviors. Many of those children were severely impaired and would spend their time flapping their hands, spinning or rocking, and making high-pitched sounds. Some children might show some improvement over time, but in general, they were profoundly impaired. The children demonstrated no interest in people; their attraction was to objects. Kanner named the condition "infantile autism."

Kanner recognized the syndrome as a developmental disorder that pervaded many, if not all, areas of the child's life. As a result, it came to be a part of that group of conditions referred to as the

PDDs. For many years, the diagnosis of autism in the U.S. was based on Kanner's criteria.

Hans Asperger's Contribution

During the 1980s in England, Dr. Lorna Wing, a British psychiatrist whose daughter had been diagnosed with autism, became interested in the work of Hans Asperger, an Austrian pediatrician. Dr. Asperger had published a dissertation in which he wrote about a group of young boys who were described as being "little professors" because of their obsession with a subject area, often unusual and restrictive in nature. These children were described as having difficulty with communication, problems with social relationships, and an inability to understand others' state of mind.

In one of those curious coincidences often seen in science, Dr. Asperger wrote his paper in the 1940s, in the same time frame as when Kanner was writing his influential work in the United States. Dr. Kanner's work was published in major scientific journals and

---

THE MEANING OF "AUTISM"

Autism is a Greek word for "self." The children who Dr. Leo Kanner observed had no interest in others, and Kanner used the word "autism" to refer to the children's withdrawal into their own world.

became well known. Asperger's work was written in German and published in an obscure journal during World War II. As a result, it was virtually unknown in the English-speaking world until Dr. Wing called attention to it.

Lorna Wing's Contribution

Dr. Lorna Wing recognized the similarity of the two conditions and suggested that they may represent different degrees of the same underlying impairment. Dr. Uta Frith, another researcher from the U.K., subsequently translated the Asperger paper into English, making it accessible to other researchers. Work on integrating the two diagnoses then began.

Is Autism a Spectrum Disorder?

Kanner's patients had more severe difficulties than Asperger's patients. Many were mute and unable to relate to their parents and were intellectually retarded. These patients were likely to end up being institutionalized for life. Others demonstrated some improvement but never caught up with their peers in terms of development. Asperger's patients were more verbal and, while eccentric, better functioning. But both groups shared the same triad of difficulties: difficulty with communication, difficulty with social relationships, and the inability to read others' state of mind. The idea that this might be a spectrum of disorders ranging from Kanner's very severely disturbed children to the higher-functioning children with AS, began to develop. The concept of an autism spectrum guides most thinking and research today.

Open Issues About AS and Autism

Many unresolved questions remain about the nature of AS and autism and whether there really is a spectrum or continuous range of autistic disorders. There are ongoing attempts to better understand all of these conditions and to refine the diagnostic criteria as more information is acquired. This is critically important in order to conduct much-needed research into the causes of the disorder.

Simon Baron-Cohen, a Cambridge University–based AS researcher, offers an interesting, if controversial, perspective. Dr. Baron-Cohen suggests that individuals at the highest end of the spectrum are demonstrating what might be called "extreme male behavior," and he invites us to be curious about where normal ends and impairment begins.

A Valuable Natural Difference

Dr. Baron-Cohen's view of AS as an extreme variant of "normal" behavior is shared by a number of those who have AS. Many individuals with AS argue that this condition should not be seen as an impairment but rather as a natural variant of the human condition. They point out that the nature of this variant contributes to an ability to focus that is less likely to occur in NTs and that this capacity for intense focus often results in unique solutions to difficult problems.

The Genius Gene

A number of people believe that many individuals who have made remarkable contributions to society (for example, Albert Einstein) likely have AS. Some adults with AS take this as evidence that this

DR. TEMPLE GRANDIN

The work of Dr. Temple Grandin is frequently cited as an example of the valuable contributions made by those on the autism spectrum. Dr. Grandin was diagnosed as autistic as a child and has become probably the most famous autistic person in the world, writing and lecturing globally. She has leveraged her capacity for intense focus and her particular way of thinking to design extremely effective and humane ways of handling beef cattle in stockyards. Dr. Grandin attributes her success in large part to her ability to focus and see details that NTs miss.

condition is not only a variant of normal but may be a form of genius that is important to the future of the human species.

The Painful Side of AS

It is clear from work with adults with AS and the NTs who interact with them that these differences, however they are characterized, often result in much pain and anguish. Dr. Tony Attwood, an expert who has spent his career writing and lecturing extensively about AS, discusses the AS-NT relationship as one where the individuals come from different cultures. He describes his role in working with AS-NT couples as that of a translator. Dr. Attwood helps each individual to understand and respect the other's way of thinking and being.

Barbara Jacobs, a British author, writes very powerfully and sympathetically of her own painful experience of being in a relationship with a man with AS. In her book, *Loving Mr. Spock,* she describes the two conditions of AS and NT as "parallel universes." She writes of her discovery of AS and reports how it helped her to gain some understanding of that other universe. It also became the means by which she and her partner negotiated some of the difficulties of the relationship.

The Prevalence of AS

If we examine the estimates of the number of people with AS, we can see that the number of encounters between individuals with AS and those who are neurotypical is anything but trivial. Analysis of prevalence rates shows ranges from 1 in 1,000 to 1 in 250 people. Many experts believe that the above numbers underestimate the real figure because of the many people who remain undiagnosed.

A Growing Problem

The number of people diagnosed with AS is growing, in some cases at an astonishing rate. In 1999, California Health and Human Services conducted a study that compared the populations receiving services for autism disorders in 1987 with those receiving services in 1998. During that eleven-year time period, the number of people receiving services for autism (including AS) increased 210 percent. Autism without mental retardation (that is AS) showed the largest increase.

There is disagreement about these dramatic increases in the occurrence of autistic disorders and what they mean. Some argue that it is just a matter of better knowledge of the condition, resulting in more identified cases. Others dismiss it as the diagnosis *du jour.* But many experts in the field express their concern that something as yet unknown is triggering a dramatic increase in incidence. These are serious concerns, and, fortunately, many more researchers are working to understand them, using new tools such as fMRI (functional magnetic resonance imaging, a means of scanning activity in the living brain), genetic studies, and other research methods.

The Search for Help

If there is an actual increase in the number of people with AS or autism spectrum disorders, there will be a need to have enough clinicians trained to recognize the condition and to work with individuals on the autism spectrum. This brings us to a very practical issue. Our clinical experience and much contact with others interested in this area indicate that it is difficult to get an accurate diagnosis, especially for individuals who are high functioning, or the most able adults. Many clinicians, whether psychiatrists, psychologists, or social workers, are unaware of AS or think of it only as a child's diagnosis. As mentioned earlier, AS is a relatively new diagnosis first included in the DSM-IV-R in 1994. For many currently practicing professionals, it was not part of their training, and they may not be familiar with it.

The Danger of Misdiagnosis

We know that many with AS who seek professional help are misdiagnosed. In part, this is probably due to professionals who lack experience with the syndrome. In other cases, the diagnostic criteria for certain personality disorders (longstanding personality traits that cause difficulty for the individual or those around them) overlap with characteristics of AS. For example, the diagnosis of schizoid personality is based on social withdrawal and odd thinking. Some individuals with AS are frequently with-

'REFRIGERATOR MOTHERS'

Although Kanner's autism was part of the training curricula in most graduate programs for many years, because there were few means to treat it, it did not receive much attention. Treatment with medications or psychoanalytic (talk therapy) treatment approaches were not effective, so little emphasis was given to autism or the other PDDs. Thinking at that time put a lot of emphasis on the mother-child relationship. Mothers of autistic children who did seek help were frequently told that the child's problem was a result of their coldness; this was the origin of the now discredited term "refrigerator mother."

drawn, and their thinking may seem odd because of their literal use of words. Another diagnosis that might be confused with AS is narcissistic personality disorder. To make the diagnosis of narcissistic personality disorder, the individual must behave in ways that are self-centered and must lack empathy for others. The nature of AS thinking means that individuals with AS have problems understanding another person's state of mind and that they have difficulty seeing others' points of view, a set of characteristics that, if the examiner is not knowledgeable about AS, might lead to the misdiagnosis of narcissistic personality.

Another misdiagnosis given to individuals with AS is schizophrenia. An individual with AS uses language very literally and if asked, "Do you hear voices?" may respond "yes," meaning that the person can hear others speak. In a clinical setting, this may be interpreted as hearing voices that are not real, and the person may be given a diagnosis of a serious mental illness.

Clinicians have noted that the two personality disorders, schizoid and narcissistic, generally do not respond to standard methods of treatment such as medications, insight-oriented talk therapy, or psychoanalysis. If the actual diagnosis is AS, it would not be surprising if those treatments did not work. AS is not responsive to those kinds of interventions, primarily because it is a hardwired neurobiological condition that involves differences in the way the individual thinks and relates to the world.

False-Negative Diagnosis

In addition to misdiagnosis, individuals with AS, who have lived with feeling different all their lives, when seeking professional

OVERCOMING MISDIAGNOSIS

Wendy Lawson, author of the book *Build Your Own Life,* was misdiagnosed with schizophrenia for over twenty-five years. When she was finally correctly diagnosed as having AS, she set about writing a book that was written with the intent of helping others with AS learn to manage their lives. She is truly an inspirational example of someone who struggled to overcome a misdiagnosis for many years. She has gone on to make a very real contribution to furthering the understanding of AS through her writings and lectures.

help to understand their problem may be told by clinicians unfamiliar with the diagnosis, or only familiar with its most severe presentation, that there is nothing wrong with them (known as a "false-negative" diagnosis). Unfortunately, this false-negative diagnosis may result in denial of the right intervention or services that would improve life for the person with AS and those around him or her. Not only is the adult with AS done a disservice; significant others will be left to struggle with bewilderment and hurt because they will not have an understanding of AS-NT differences.

Lauri, a thirty-five-year-old woman, had been in a very stressful relationship with a man, now her fiancé, whom she loved deeply for his kindness and intelligence. After reading about the condition, she recognized that AS could be the explanation for so many of the behaviors that caused so much difficulty in their relationship. Her fiancé readily agreed to have an evaluation. He had a lifelong history of problems with interpersonal relationships and did not understand why, since he tried hard to be kind. Frank sought a consultation with a clinician who, after one meeting, assured him that he did not have AS—and said that AS was a diagnosis for children. The mental health professional suggested that his girlfriend might need help—that she was too sensitive. In typical, logical AS fashion, Frank felt that this meeting proved that he did not have a problem. He no longer had any motivation to change and felt that Lauri's upsets were just a result of her oversensitivity. After much soul searching, Lauri finally left the relationship. She continued to mourn the loss two years later.

Summing It All Up

You are probably wondering why so much emphasis is put on the diagnosis of AS, its history, and the concern about finding someone qualified to diagnose it. It is because diagnosis is the single most critical element in finding solutions to living with Asperger Syndrome.

Once the diagnosis is made, and the adult with AS accepts it, the process of gaining understanding can begin. Armed with the knowledge that AS is a neurobiological difference that affects the way the person with AS deals with the world, the adult with AS can begin the work of defining those differences. And in just the same way that we become more effective in a new country as we learn about the culture, learning about AS and the AS differences will allow us to develop new ways to communicate and relate more effectively.

CHAPTER TWO

The Importance of Diagnosis and Misdiagnosis

"Asperger Syndrome? That's the problem? I've never heard of it!" stated Annie, a pretty nineteen-year-old college student. Annie had come to my office with her mother, Maureen, several weeks earlier. Maureen was worried because Annie's complaints of depression and anxiety were "worse than usual." Although Annie was doing okay at a local county college, she wanted to drop out of school. Annie had chosen to leave a prestigious university her freshman year because of problems getting along with other students.

Maureen was very concerned. "Annie has become more withdrawn. She is staying in her room on the computer for days at a time." Maureen wanted Annie to see a therapist. Annie agreed but insisted she would only see a therapist if her mother came along.

I asked Annie if she would like to talk alone, but she refused. She seemed unable to begin to tell me her story, so I asked Maureen what she was worried about. She said, "Annie frequently says that she wishes she was dead. I am afraid Annie might commit suicide."

At this point, Annie interrupted. "The problem isn't me and isn't schoolwork; it's the other kids. They are mean to me." I asked how they were mean. "They say mean things like that the things I am interested in are boring. They don't listen to me. Sometimes they interrupt or walk away." She said they don't invite her to lunch, or they go to a place they know she won't go because she can't stand the noise.

Maureen said that this pattern of having trouble making friends started back when Annie was a small child. Playmates would stop coming for play dates because Annie needed the play to be according to her rules. She would throw a tantrum if the other kids changed things. Maureen became tearful and apologetic, saying she knew it sounded like she was a poor mother and that she couldn't manage her child, but that no matter how she tried, Annie would become upset. She said she had been trying for years to help Annie with social situations, but now that she was an adult, Annie had become resentful of her help.

At that point, Annie began talking over her mother about some computer game characters. It seemed likely that her mother's crying and our talking about Annie's difficulties with people were triggering Annie's anxiety. Annie was trying to change the conversation to her special interest—the computer game characters the other kids had outgrown and now called boring. Annie was obsessed by these characters and felt comfortable talking about them. It was also her way of keeping her mother from talking about these upsetting things. I asked Annie what was upsetting her. "I am not upset. My mother treats me like a baby."

Over a period of several weeks, Annie became more comfortable and was willing to talk about what was happening at school. We had worked out some strategies to help her deal better with other students, and she was pleased. It was while we were talking about this that she suddenly asked me about her diagnosis. She said, "I've decided I want to learn more about why I am different."

The Importance of a Diagnosis
Getting a Diagnosis

Making a diagnosis is a significant act that must be taken seriously. It is the responsibility of the one doing the diagnosing to make every effort to be sure that the diagnosis is within the scope of his or her expertise. If this is not the case, the only ethical thing to do is to refer the individual to a more competent resource.

Dr. Stephan Behnke reminds us in the *Monitor on Psychology* that a diagnosis has clinical, personal, and social significance. Clinically, the diagnosis defines the condition and the correct treatment or intervention. An incorrect diagnosis or failure to make a diagnosis when the condition is present (referred to as a "false-negative" diagnosis) means that the individual will get the

∽∾

AN IMPORTANT NOTE TO READERS

The issue of seeking a diagnosis is both a crucial and sensitive one. It can't be stressed too much that getting a diagnosis is critical to finding solutions to living with AS. This book is based on the premise that the person with AS has been accurately diagnosed, has accepted the diagnosis, and now wants to develop more understanding of the condition.

wrong treatment or, in the case of the false-negative diagnosis, be denied treatment. At a personal level, the diagnosis becomes a part of how the person feels about himself or herself. In many cases, people with Asperger Syndrome (AS) have always known there was something different about them, and the diagnosis of their problem helps their "different-ness" finally make sense. For other people, it may initially be difficult to integrate the diagnosis into their image of themselves, but without it, the person with AS is denied the correct treatment or services to which he or she may be entitled. As a result, the person may continue to have difficulties that he or she has no way of resolving. At the social level, a diagnosis opens the way to more acceptance of unusual or different behavior and encourages the seeking of services, such as counseling, that may improve the individual's life.

The Value of a Diagnosis

There is agreement in the autism spectrum disorders community that it is critical for children to be diagnosed as early in life as possible. The younger the brain, the more it is able to respond to input designed to increase its internal connectivity. This in turn may improve certain skills relating to improved communication and better functioning, especially of a social nature.

In a striking number of instances, the diagnosis of an AS adult comes about as the result of the evaluation and diagnosis of a child in the family. There has been a marked increase in awareness of early childhood disorders. As a result, more children are being identified as having difficulties and are referred for assessment to determine if they need special services. As the parents participate in the evaluation, they hear the diagnostic criteria and in many cases recognize themselves, or one parent hears the criteria and realizes that his or her spouse has some of the same traits. Some individuals identified in this way will go on to be evaluated. Others will choose not to have an evaluation. However, thoughtful clinicians recognize that the diagnosis of an autistic spectrum disorder in the family has very broad-reaching effects, including the possible identification of other family members as being on the spectrum. It is important for the professional community to make sure that the family is aware of and can gain access to clinicians who work with adults with AS if the family needs it.

In the case of adults with AS, clinical experience tells us that individuals with AS differ in their opinion about the value of a diagnosis. Some have no interest in being diagnosed for what they see as a mind difference rather than a problem. Other AS adults, who have always felt different or unable to fit in, are very relieved to get a diagnosis and find out more about what they have been struggling with all their lives. They see the diagnosis as a path to being able to manage their lives better.

Wendy Lawson, who was diagnosed with AS as an adult, has written a very positive self-help book for individuals with AS titled *Building Your Own Life*. Wendy tells of having struggled with feelings of anxiety and confusion for as long as she can remember. She was misdiagnosed with schizophrenia for twenty-five years. During that time, she was hospitalized a number of times and was given powerful drugs that only made her problem worse. When she was finally given the correct diagnosis of AS, she began conducting research to understand the diagnosis. Wendy discovered the differences in the way adults with AS and NTs think and relate to the world. Over time, she developed many coping skills to help her deal with her AS, and she shares those in her book. Before the correct diagnosis, Wendy had no way of understanding the condition with which she was struggling or of finding ways to improve her life. After getting the correct diagnosis, she has gained success as an author and worldwide lecturer on AS. Her work is a testimony to her ability to reach out and engage others with AS, or those with AS in their midst, with a life-affirming attitude.

Resisting a Diagnosis

Others with AS resist or are not interested in seeking a diagnosis. This seems to be particularly true in older individuals. Perhaps they feel that a diagnosis will make no difference in their lives, so what would be the point? Unfortunately, this often means that the person continues to struggle with communication and relationships. In other cases, work with AS-NT couples indicates that if the AS partner in a committed relationship has been diagnosed with AS and denies the diagnosis, the relationship almost always ends.

Diagnosis and Significant Others
AS is a hidden condition. There are few or no physical signs that would suggest that the adult with AS functions differently from NTs. It is when individuals with AS are not able to function and manage their life or when those with AS and NTs are in situations where they must interact with one another that the difficulties in communication and social interaction become obvious. When this is the case, the differences that occur, and the problems that result, are usually misinterpreted on both sides. The NT may see the behavior of the individual with AS as rude or callous, while the individual with AS may feel rejected for no reason. Without a diagnosis, the individuals do not understand that there are differences in brain wiring. Anger, resentment, confusion, and disappointment develop, putting the relationship at risk. If the diagnosis is known, the source of tensions becomes understandable and the parties can engage in seeking solutions to work through the problems.

Diagnosis in Children
Parents of children with AS have stated that the "invisible" quality of the diagnosis can make it more stressful to raise their kids.

Overstimulating situations, changes in routine, or other occasions that become too much for the AS child to cope with frequently result in meltdowns, the name given to the intense emotional upset that the child experiences. To an observer, it looks like the child is having a temper tantrum. If a parent gives in to the child to cut short a scene, people who see this often think the child is undisciplined and is getting away with bad behavior. These types of situations make the parent's already difficult job even more painful.

Making the Choice to Seek a Diagnosis

Unlike children who have parents who often desperately search to find a diagnosis to help them understand their child's differences, for an adult, the decision to seek a diagnosis is voluntary. It may be very hard for NTs to accept that fact if they believe that someone they care about has AS, but any form of coercion, such as threats, whether by a spouse, a parent, or some authority figure, will almost certainly be resented. If the person does keep an appointment made by an NT, he will come into the office angry and unwilling to cooperate. These circumstances make a thoughtful, thorough evaluation difficult or impossible. If the therapist chooses to attempt the assessment despite the situation, there is every chance that the diagnosis will be denied by the individual with AS, and the opportunity to get help for the problem will likely be lost.

The Purpose of Diagnosing

The word "diagnosis" comes from a Greek word meaning to know. Simply put, to know something is the beginning of understanding it. When we know about something, we give it a name in order to be able to talk about it and to learn about. And that is the first of three purposes of making a diagnosis—to give a name to a condition and to provide information about it and its cause. The second purpose is to tell us the prognosis, or to put it differently, the course and likely outcome of a condition. Finally, a diagnosis gives us access to what is known about treatment or interventions.

The First Function of Diagnosis—Naming the Condition

A diagnosis gives us a name for the condition that helps us understand it. It tells us what a condition is, based on an existing body of knowledge. It also provides information on what the problem is not. For example, the diagnosis of AS tells us that it is not a mental illness.

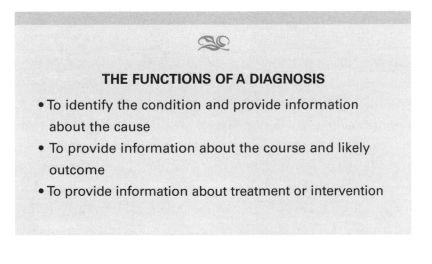

THE FUNCTIONS OF A DIAGNOSIS

• To identify the condition and provide information about the cause
• To provide information about the course and likely outcome
• To provide information about treatment or intervention

The Value of a Diagnosis to an Adult with AS
In providing a diagnosis, by giving a name to a condition, we've taken the first step toward being able to manage it. For individuals with AS, many who have struggled with the feeling that they are different all their lives, the fact that the difference has a name, and that others understand it, often comes as a huge relief. A part of that relief is knowing that they are not alone—that others have the same condition. For many, a diagnosis often ends the terrible sense of isolation that they have experienced.

As AS has become better known to the general public, a number of newspapers have carried stories about the relief experienced by people with AS when they have discovered the name for their condition. A *New York Times* article described the reaction of a forty-nine-year-old man who had felt different and isolated for as long as he could remember. In his reading, he came across a description of AS. He immediately recognized that it described his own lifelong painful differences. His moving story described the relief he felt simply by knowing what his problem was.

The Value of a Diagnosis to Significant Others
It is not only the person with AS who may benefit from and be greatly relieved by a diagnosis. As described earlier, AS is a pervasive developmental disorder that affects many aspects of the individual's life. Adults with AS process information, communicate, and relate to others differently than NTs do. These differences are often experienced by NTs as rudeness or a lack of caring and cause pain to those NTs around the individual with AS. Having a diagnosis that explains the source of these behaviors becomes a

valuable explanation and is often the foundation for dealing with the behavior in constructive ways.

David and Catherine are having problems in their marriage. "Catherine refuses to allow my parents to come to our house. They are devastated." David, twenty-five, along with his parents, operate a florist business. They have always been a close family. He and Catherine married three years ago. Besides being unwilling to see David's parents, Catherine has also become more and more unwilling to see friends. "She is obsessed with decorating the house. Ever since she visited that historic home several years ago, all she wants to do or to talk about is decorating. She took a bunch of pictures of the interior. She spends many hours and more money than we can afford compulsively searching for stuff to duplicate what she saw in that house." I asked Catherine why she wasn't comfortable with David's parents visiting. She said, "David's father won't let me talk about decorating and keeps trying to change the subject. David's mother wants to take over and decorate my house." She felt that her in-laws treated her like a child. David was stunned. He said the interactions he had seen between his wife and parents did not match his wife's reports. David said, "My parents are interested in Catherine's decorating, but my dad likes to talk about other things, too. Catherine's not interested in anything except her decorating." David said he felt that his mother's questions, which Catherine interpreted as criticism and telling her what to do, were attempts to build a relationship with her daughter-in-law based on the only subject Catherine was interested in talking about. It became clear after several sessions that Catherine had AS. She agreed to a consultation at a well-known academic center and was diagnosed with AS. She had no curiosity about the syndrome, stating only that she had "always been this way." Her husband researched the syndrome in depth. He was concerned about the impact of AS on their relationship but was relieved to understand that there was a reason for his wife's behavior. When last seen, he reported that he was working hard to understand his wife.

The Second Function of Diagnosis—To Provide Information
The second purpose of a diagnosis is to provide information about the likely course of the syndrome and its outcome. AS is a relatively recently recognized syndrome. It was first identified in children, and it was not considered that the condition continued into adulthood. As a result, there was no research for a time about its impact throughout the lifespan. However, as AS was better understood, awareness grew that it did not disappear in adulthood. As people with AS mature, many learn ways to compensate, making the condition less obvious. But the fact that individuals with AS learn to compensate does not mean that the condition goes away. Books written by adults with AS, who have generously shared their personal stories, give us a meaningful way to understand and appreciate the impact of AS in adulthood and the effort required to compensate. A good example is Liane Holliday Willey' book, *Pretending to Be Normal*, which includes a moving personal account of her experience living with AS.

RECOGNIZING A CONDITION IN CHILDHOOD FIRST

It is not unusual for a condition to first be recognized in children. Attention deficit disorder (ADD) is another example of a diagnosis that was first noted in children, and only later did we understand that ADD was not outgrown and that it did not disappear in adulthood. Because it was recognized that this is a lifelong disorder, a great many adults have benefited by having their diagnosis recognized, understood, and treated.

AS Across the Lifespan

The identification of AS as a pervasive developmental disorder provides us with important information about the course of the condition across the lifespan. We know that it is hardwired into the brain and that it starts very early in life, if not before birth. We also know that its process and outcome are influenced by a number of variables. Perhaps the most critical variable is IQ level. Those with greater intellectual endowment tend to fare better across the lifespan than those less intellectually endowed. It also seems certain that environment and opportunity play a large role in the prognosis. Supportive, highly interactive environments ensure that the individual will have the greatest opportunity to reach his or her potential.

Eustacia Cutler, Temple Grandin's mother, writes in her book, *A Thorn in My Pocket,* of her commitment to creating an environment for Temple that would keep her actively, deeply engaged with the world (for more on Temple Grandin, see page 35 in Chapter One). Temple's abilities have developed to the point that she was able to complete her doctorate and become an expert in her chosen field. Temple's mother's sensitive appreciation of Temple, not as an autistic but as a unique individual with her own interesting personality and talent, no doubt played a large role in Temple's success. Her insistence on Temple being involved with the family and the world around her and her careful choice of educational opportunities for her daughter has helped Temple to have a successful life.

The Third Function of Diagnosis—Defining Treatment

We are early in the identification of the most beneficial treatments for AS, especially AS in adults. Research shows that in AS, there are significant differences in the brain and its circuitry from very early in life. These differences are probably responsible for the differences in the way adults with AS approach the world. Although it will not benefit those who are now adults, there is much research effort underway to find a way to identify AS as early as possible in infancy. The very young brain is more plastic, meaning it is more easily altered by certain experiences. The hope is that early interventions will influence the development of neurons in the brain in a way that will make it easier for people with AS to navigate their way through life.

Centers of excellence in autism spectrum research, such as the Yale Child Study Center, anticipate using technology such as fMRI (functional magnetic resonance imaging) to study the impact of early intervention on the developing brain. fMRI is a technology that allows researchers to take scans of activity in the living brain. It is believed that the earlier the child with AS is diagnosed, the more effective therapy will be, because the child's brain is still developing. Taking repeated fMRI scans over time while the child is being treated will give us information about the effectiveness of the treatment.

Misdiagnosis: Why It Happens and the Consequences
AS Is Not Yet Widely Known or Understood

Perhaps the most common reason for misdiagnosis (or no diagnosis) is the lack of clinicians familiar with the syndrome for reasons previously discussed. This is particularly true for adults seeking a diagnosis. There is also reluctance on the part of some clinicians to label an adult with a developmental disorder, particularly if in many ways the adult is high functioning. Unfortunately, this usually means that the individual is deprived of a true understanding of his or her problem and is left without a meaningful treatment plan or even a means of communicating to significant others the nature of his or her problems. For people who are in a relationship with undiagnosed or incorrectly diagnosed individuals with AS, there are problems as well. They are left to deal with frustrating, mystifying behavior with no clue as to the nature of the problem or what to do about it.

Karen Rodman, founder of FAAAS (Families of Adults Afflicted with Asperger Syndrome), a resource Web site for information about adult AS as well as a support group for people with adults with AS in their lives, has shared with many the couple's long and painful journey to get an accurate diagnosis of Karen's husband's condition. Karen and her husband spent many years seeking help for their problems. Despite her having a detailed diary of the kinds of behaviors that were so stressful in their marriage, she was unable to get mental health professionals to recognize her husband's difficulties and to see the impact on her and on their marriage. Time after time she was told that his actions were "just normal male behavior" and that she was too sensitive. Karen was told several times that she should either accept it or leave and divorce. During that long, frustrating search, Karen was told repeatedly that the problem was hers. She was prescribed powerful drugs that only made things worse. Finally, in 1996, after ten years of visits to mental health professionals by herself and her husband, they were told by a Boston neuropsychiatrist that her husband had both AS and Tourettes syndrome. Tourettes is an involuntary tic movement disorder that is often seen with AS. Karen describes the enormous relief she felt when she finally understood the reason for her distress over the years. It became the starting point for rebuilding her relationship with her husband, based on a new understanding.

Diagnosis Problems Are Too Familiar

Autism spectrum Web sites overflow with the frustration of parents of adults with AS as well as spouses of undiagnosed people with AS who have recognized that there is something different or odd in the behavior they see but who have been told there is nothing wrong. Thanks to a greater investment in research, there is a growing awareness of the autism spectrum and an increase in the number of clinicians familiar with it, but it still takes some research to find clinicians who are familiar with the diagnosis in adults. It is most helpful to get a referral from someone who has been diagnosed with AS, or someone whose child has been diagnosed with AS. There are also a number of major university medical centers that have autism research centers that can be consulted.

Underserved Populations

Despite the advancement in the accurate recognition of AS in adults, there are two groups that continue to be underserved, probably because the diagnostic criteria need to be refined. These two groups are high-functioning adults and women with AS.

High-Functioning Adults

Individuals at the most able end of the autistic spectrum have the most hidden form of this disorder and, as a result, these individuals and their family are often the most disadvantaged in terms of getting a diagnosis. Because they have higher IQs, high-functioning adults are able to work out ways to compensate for their difficulties in communication or in social functioning that are based on logical reasoning. They're also likely to seek out a friend or partner who is high functioning and mimic their behaviors to manage socially. High-functioning adults also often rely on the friend or partner for social judgments about things like office politics. They may also depend on these same people to create order and structure in their lives. As a result, people will see a picture of a successful individual, in the world outside the home. Compensating for AS differences, however, comes at a very high cost in terms of effort, and many times, in the privacy of their home, adults with AS are not willing or able to make the considerable effort that it would take to function as well there as they do at work or out in the world. As a result, the families are left to deal with the consequences of the AS way of thinking and AS behaviors that can feel callous, hurtful, or controlling. Because this behavior often is seen only in the home, it is very important to have information not only from the individual with AS but also from those who interact with him or her at home.

Seeking Input from Others
The need for input from significant others can be a problem in some cases. Mental health professionals are not used to seeking input from family members when they are working with adult patients. In addition, our medical system is rooted in doctor/patient confidentiality, so the doctor must get the patient's permission to allow the clinician to include family members in the diagnostic process. Because it is also common for people with AS to misperceive their circumstances because of the differences in the way their minds work, their self-reports can be unreliable. For example, not understanding how certain behaviors can be hurtful to NTs, they only register the NT reaction and as a result see the NT as the "one with the problem." Finally, adults

with AS function best when they are in a structured situation, such as a clinical interview, so the difficulties that they can experience in ordinary life will probably not show up in the clinical setting. All of these factors complicate making or getting an accurate diagnosis in the case of AS. One of the most important steps that adults who suspect they might have AS can take to ensure an accurate diagnosis is to make sure that a significant other(s) is included in the diagnostic process.

Women with AS

It's been thought for a long time by those working in the area of AS that males with AS outnumber females; the most frequently quoted ratio is 4:1. But in more recent years, many clinicians who have a lot of experience working with AS, such as Dr. Tony Attwood, a leading AS expert from Australia, believe that women with AS may be an underdiagnosed population. As has happened in other medical conditions such as heart disease, the AS diagnostic criteria have been developed with a mostly male population. We also don't know, for example, if females with AS present with certain behaviors in their profile that are different from those of males. We don't know if there are certain gender-related behaviors that might cause us to miss the diagnosis. Our culture defines the gender differences that shape the way we are socialized from a very young age. For example, there is a lot more pressure on female children than on male children to conform to social rules. It is likely that AS women are indoctrinated from an early age to adopt more conforming behavior and to behave less aggressively than their male counterparts.

'RULE ENFORCERS'

We know that individuals with AS are predisposed to follow rules. In fact, their insistence on following rules themselves and trying to enforce the rules on others is often a cause for their being ostracized as children. They are the self-appointed rule enforcers, or as the other kids see it, the kid who tattles to the teacher. We can assume that if society demands more conformity in females, young females with AS will probably internalize those rules. And in fact, in her book about raising her autistic daughter, Temple Drandin, Eustacia Cutler remembers Temple's insistence on wearing scratchy, stiff petticoats to Sunday church services. Temple would wear these petticoats even though they caused her extreme discomfort (her sensory problems made her skin very sensitive). When Temple was asked why she wore the petticoats, she responded, "because that is what you are supposed to do."

Women and Aggression

Aggression is tolerated more often in males than in females. The frustration those with AS experience because of difficulties in communication can result in feelings of anger and aggression. This is more likely to be acted out by males with AS than by females with AS. The social pressure on females with AS to not be aggressive may lead to their turning anger and aggressive feelings inward, resulting in their being depressed or behaving passive-aggressively. Passive-aggressive behavior is behavior where anger is not expressed directly but is acted out in ways to make the target of the anger feel angry and frustrated.

Liz and her daughter Jenna are having problems. Liz called me and said, "It's hard to explain, but every time I turn around, Jenna and I are having problems. I am so frustrated; I don't know what to do." Jenna had recently been diagnosed as having AS; her oldest brother, Robert, had been diagnosed with autism when he was two years old. Liz described the family as very much caught up in Robert's recent move to a college setting. She said that the usual household routines were disturbed. Liz couldn't pinpoint the nature of the stress between her and Jenna. "We just keep having these upsetting incidents. I feel like I am walking on eggshells all the time; I don't know what will go wrong next."

In our first joint session, I asked Liz to describe for me a recent upsetting incident. Liz said she had been upset that morning. "I drop Jenna off at the high school every morning on my way to work. I teach in the middle school. This morning, just as she has done every morning for more than a week, Jenna disappeared into the bathroom just as we were ready to leave the house, claiming she had to use the toilet. By the time Jenna came out, I knew we were going to be late for school and work. No matter what I try, Jenna still manages to be in the bathroom when we are supposed to leave." Liz was clearly stressed and upset. She felt trapped because Jenna said she had to go to the bathroom and that she had tried to go earlier but couldn't. "Do you want me to have an accident?" she asked her mother.

It was clear that Jenna had found a way to get her mother's attention—even if it was bad attention! Jenna was angry with her mother for giving Robert all her attention. She was also having difficulty with the lack of the usual household routine. But she did not want to confront her mother directly. So instead, Jenna behaved in ways like staying in the bathroom long enough to make them late to strike out at her mother. This kind of behavior which, indirectly frustrates rather than being directly confrontational, is called passive-aggressive behavior. We talked about the disruption of the family and how it is upsetting to Jenna since she has strong needs for routine. Jenna acknowledged that, "There are too many things going on." We also talked about how much time was being devoted to Robert and that perhaps Jenna was feeling as though it was not fair— that she was not getting enough attention. Although Jenna refused to admit to being angry, the family made an effort to reestablish a routine and to pay more attention to her. Jenna's passive-aggressive behavior stopped.

As our knowledge of AS in adulthood grows, it will become easier to identify symptoms in high-functioning adults and women with AS. This will make it easier to identify the condition in these two groups.

Conditions Frequently Associated with AS

Anxiety and Depression

Most adults with AS suffer from both anxiety and depression, although to differing degrees. Because of the stress of coping with an NT world, of being unsure how to read people and understand many situations, adults with AS have to work much harder than NTs to keep their lives working well. For NTs, the innate or at least early learned ability to read a situation at a glance comes with a minimum of mental effort. For an adult with AS, each day is likely to bring new anxiety-laden situations. It has been noticed that many individuals with AS are in a state of chronic hyper-arousal, although we're not sure just why yet. Hyper-arousal is the way we feel and how our body operates when we feel threatened. Not only is this tiring, but once a person is in this hyper-aroused, or fight or flight state as it is usually referred to, he or she feels that all stakes are equally high—from facing a ferocious wild bear to having to choose a new restaurant for a family outing. In this state of high arousal, we respond to everything as if it is life-threatening. There's little wonder why people with AS experience so much anxiety!

Many people with AS, especially more high-functioning individuals, have known from very early in life that they are somehow different—that they don't fit in or feel comfortable in the NT world. This sense of isolation is often made worse when certain aspects of their condition interfere with their success in academic tasks, the world of work, or the difficult world of social relationships. They may see others around them being more successful, perhaps despite being less gifted. All too often,

66

they become depressed. In addition, individuals with AS usually do not see how their behavior affects others negatively, and this negative behavior usually results in the person with AS being rejected. They experience the rejection but do not understand the reason for it. This situation may further fuel their depression, which may become chronic. Anxiety and depression usually respond to treatment. It's important to seek help for these conditions before they become chronic.

A colleague described to me an incident that she had experienced a few years ago. My colleague had been sitting by a pool with a friend who had been diagnosed in her early twenties as having AS. The woman with AS was extremely bright and had learned to live her life quite successfully. She had never married but was a well-respected computer scientist. She watched the wind drift an empty chair float in the pool, first in one direction, then another, frequently bumping up against the wall. She said, "That chair is like me. It doesn't have any direction; it just gets bumped around in the empty pool. There is no purpose, no meaning to what happens. It just happens. Even the job I have I got by accident." My colleague said this woman's sense of depression and meaninglessness was heartbreaking.

Attention Deficit Disorder

Attention deficit disorder (ADD), especially ADD-inattentive type, is often seen in AS, although there are questions about whether this is real ADD or simply a result of the characteristics of AS that cause individuals with AS to be so focused. They may at times be so focused on something that has captured their attention that they simply do not take notice or pay attention to anything else! ADD can be responsive to the right medication in some cases, and individuals who have problems with attention and concentration should seek an evaluation from a psychiatrist to see if medication for these symptoms might be helpful.

Other Psychiatric Diagnoses
Obsessive-Compulsive Disorder
Obsessive-compulsive disorder (OCD) is frequently seen in individuals with AS and in family members of those with AS. There is not agreement whether the repetitive behaviors, such as needing possessions to be arranged in a certain order, are evidence of OCD or simply reflect the need for sameness or, said differently, the resistance by someone with AS to changes in the environment. One important difference is that in OCD, the person is anxious about the behavior and wants to stop but is unable to stop. In AS, the repetitive behavior usually has a soothing effect.

Epilepsy
Epilepsy occurs in as many as 30 percent of people with autism spectrum disorders, with the risk being much higher at the lower-functioning end of the spectrum. Individuals with AS are only slightly more at risk than the rest of the population.

Learning Disorders
Learning disorders are common in individuals with AS and in-

clude both verbal and nonverbal learning disorders. It is important that these often-coexisting conditions be identified and treated. Some are responsive to medication, and others can be helped by working with learning disorder specialists. AS also frequently impairs the ability of the individual to plan and execute more complicated tasks that require many steps. Again, work with a learning specialist can improve skills in this area. Recognizing and treating these disorders can make a great difference in the quality of life for people with AS.

Other Medical Conditions

Many individuals with AS have dietary intolerances for substances such as gluten or lactose. There is also an increased risk in AS for immune system reactions that are associated with digestive disorders such as Crohn's disease and celiac disease.

It's important to be aware of the increased risk of these medical conditions. Awareness will allow individuals with AS who might develop these conditions to take steps to get early treatment.

Summing It All Up

People with AS who choose to seek and follow up on a diagnosis are given an opportunity to learn about and to develop an appreciation for the differences in the AS and NT ways of functioning. This understanding can have a positive influence on the life of the person with AS and on his or her relationships. For NTs who live with someone with AS, the diagnosis helps them to understand why there are so many misunderstandings between them. It takes effort on both sides to understand the differences in the way those with AS and those who are NT function, but with a diagnosis, there is a roadmap that will help those with AS and those who are NT figure out how to manage their relationship. Working out better ways of relating is not easy, because it can take a while for both parties to understand how AS thinking translates into AS behavior and vice versa. Trying to work out better ways of doing things is also made harder by the resistance to change displayed by people with AS and their difficulty in generalizing what they have learned from one situation to another. But the results can be rewarding.

Finding solutions to AS begins with the syndrome being diagnosed. The diagnosis provides a new framework both for individuals with AS and for NTs to interpret what is happening between them. For people with AS, a diagnosis becomes a way to reinterpret, or reframe, their experience by looking at it from a new perspective—that of having a brain that works differently from that of NTs. This difference means that they behave in ways that are different from NTs, but these differences will now make sense. This reframing can take out a lot of the hurt that results from the frequent misunderstandings that occur between those with AS and NTs. Recognizing AS-NT differences can result in more tolerance and fewer frustrations for both groups. The more knowledge and understanding each group has of the other, the easier it is for the AS-NT cultures to interact in positive ways.

CHAPTER THREE

How We Process Information:
The Theory of Central Coherence

David and Tracy have some vacation time scheduled, and they are trying to make plans for what they will do during their time off. For the last two years, they have rented a house on a lake in Maine and invited other family members to come visit. David enjoyed these vacations and wants to rent a house again. Tracy, however, definitely does not want to rent a vacation house ever again. Her memories of the last couple of vacations are not pleasant. But, she and her husband David (who has AS), have been trying to improve their communication and understanding of one another. So Tracy decides that she should ask David why he feels as he does.

"What did you like so much about the Maine vacation?" she asks David. "Well, I liked having my coffee and cereal out on the porch every morning, and I liked my brother and his wife being there. I remember we had all my favorite foods for dinner; the first night we had steak, baked potato, and peach pie and ice cream for dessert. Then the next night, we had salmon and rice and asparagus. Then on Wednesday...." Tracy interrupts him. "Are you going to ask what the vacation was like for me?" David starts to continue his recall of their menus. He loves food and he likes to talk about what they have for meals, but Tracy holds up her hand, indicating for him to stop. "I want to tell you what last year's vacation was like for me. We got there at 3:15 in the afternoon after driving for six hours. I worked for three hours getting the house ready and beds made. Then I had to go to the market for food. I fixed dinner for nine people. I was exhausted. I spent my whole vacation working, and I hated it. I don't want to do that this year."

Tracy's unhappiness and her dismay at having to do so much work on her vacation had not registered with David. He didn't understand why Tracy didn't want to go back to Maine. He wasn't comfortable going to new places and wanted to go somewhere that was familiar. David hadn't recognized Tracy's feelings when they were on the vacation, so her feelings weren't a part of his memory. He had no way to understand what she was talking about in the present conversation. David's memory of the vacation was a set of details that consisted mostly of what he had done, what they had eaten, and who was there. David, because of his AS, doesn't usually register certain kinds of information, especially people's feelings. And, he doesn't pull information together in a way that would allow him to have seen that Tracy was so unhappy on the trip.

When Tracy brought up how upset she had been on the vacation, David was surprised. He had no idea that she had hated a vacation that he had liked so much.

Tracy and David agreed on certain facts about the vacation. Sure, they were in Maine, they did have family visiting, and steak, baked potatoes, and peach pie with ice cream were served for dinner. But David's memories were of the details of the situation. The details were accurate, and clearly they were vivid for him. But Tracy's hard work and how tired and resentful she felt had not registered with David. People with Asperger Syndrome (AS) don't usually register other people's feelings, and because David did not take in Tracy's feelings, her feelings were not a part of the way he remembered the vacation. When Tracy remembered the trip, she had a more global picture or big picture. Tracy's recall of the details of each meal wasn't accurate like David's, but Tracy's memory included information that was not part of David's memory. She remembered how tiring the drive up to the lake was and that she was exhausted even before she got started making the house ready for them and their guests. She remembered having to shop for all of David's favorite food, and most of all, she remembered how tired and frustrated she was with all the work she had to do. She kept thinking, why doesn't David see it's supposed to be my vacation, too? Tracy's mind puts together information from both internal and external sources. She remembered the things that had happened, and she also remembered how unhappy she felt. Tracy used this information to put together a whole picture of the vacation, rather than to just focus on the details the way David did. Thinking about that big picture, she realized that she did not ever want to take another vacation like that.

Both David and Tracy were describing accurately what they each remembered about the vacation, but their memories of the vacation are very different. David's AS thinking meant he was focused on the details of the vacation. He did not see a big picture. Tracy's memories for the details were not as clear, but she was very aware of the big picture and how renting a vacation place is too much work. Seeing things very differently is frequently the case between NTs and those with AS because of the differences in the way people with AS and those who are NT see and register information. It's easy to see these differences when we look at David's and Tracy's memories of the vacation. These same kinds of differences occur much of the time when people with AS and NTs have interactions. The type of information gathered, how that information registers, and how the individuals process that information means they usually have a lot of difficulty understanding one another.

Frequently, when people hear an NT-AS story such as Tracy and David's, there is a tendency to dismiss it as just being "typical male behavior." It is not typical male behavior. The critical difference is that non-AS males have the ability to see the situation; they can both see and understand why the other person is unhappy. For a person with AS, emotional information—the way the other person feels—can be invisible. Or if the person with AS does see an emotional reaction such as frustration, he or she doesn't interpret it correctly. The person with AS is not intentionally ignoring the other person's feelings or deliberately not paying attention to the other's stress. The other person's feelings do not register, or they register only with great effort, and even then it is difficult for the person with AS to understand another's feelings. A typical NT male is able to be aware of and understand other's feelings if he wants to. He has the choice of letting feelings register with him if he chooses to. This is not the case in individuals with AS.

Some people with AS, as they gain life experience, become more aware of others' feelings and thoughts, but they process them in a different part of their brain than NT individuals do. Probably for this reason, understanding other's thoughts and feelings never comes in the easy, natural way it does with NTs and often fails when the individual with AS is stressed or in an emotional situation.

AS-NT Cognitive Differences

Cognition refers to the way we know things. Our cognitive style includes the way we learn, think, and imagine things, as well as remember things. Understanding the differences in cognitive style between NTs and people with AS is fundamental to understanding the two cultures and the problems they have in interacting.

While there is some variability among NTs in their preference for global or "big picture" thinking versus paying attention to details, overall, NTs have a strong need to put their experience together in a way that lets them make sense of it or get the gist of it. Details are often less important to an NT than gaining an understanding of the whole situation, and NTs often lose track of details if they don't seem important to the meaning of what's happening. For example, NTs may not remember whether they had oat cereal or corn flakes this morning, but they are very likely to recall the fact that they had breakfast with their boss!

Getting the Gist of It

"He can't see the forest for the trees" is a slang way of saying that a person is so caught up in the details of something that he is not getting the gist of it or what is really important about the situation. Gist, a word that is important in our discussion of cognitive styles, means pulling information together in a way that allows us to understand a higher meaning. To explain what this means, imagine that someone said to you, "You are going to get into trouble for that." Depending on what the situation is, that statement can have very different implications. If, for example, the person saying it is a good friend, and you are just fooling around, you will know she is just kidding and keep on with what you are doing. But, if the person saying it is a police officer at the scene of an automobile accident, and he says it in a very serious voice, you'll hear the words and respond very differently. You'll stop whatever you are doing or try to explain why you are doing it.

The decision to handle the two situations—the one with your friend and the other with the police officer—differently is based on your getting the gist of the situation. Gist refers to figuring out the meaning of all the aspects of the situation not just the words you hear: "You are going to get in trouble." When you are looking for the gist of something, you will call to mind information that you know that will help you to judge the situation. For example, if you know that your friend likes to kid you (information from your memory), and you are aware that the activity you are doing is harmless (has no negative consequences), and you note your friend's tone of voice and smile (looking and hearing), you have pulled together information from the situation and added in additional information from your mind to gain an understanding of the situation. By putting all this information together, it is clear to you that you don't have to take what she is saying seriously. Because you have figured out the gist of the situation—that your friend is just teasing you and there is no risk—you know that you can continue to do what you are doing.

In the situation with the police officer, you know that an automobile accident is taken seriously (from knowledge or past experience), you are aware that the police officer has authority over you in this situation (the law), and you know he is serious from his tone of voice and the look on his face (looking and hearing). Pulling all this information from different sources, internal and external, together in your mind allows you to understand and judge the situation as being serious. Your understanding of the situation tells you how to respond appropriately. This higher-level meaning is what is meant by gist.

What Is the Drive for Central Coherence?

The drive for central coherence is the ability to recognize the relevance of different types of knowledge or information to a particular situation and to put these things together in a way that allows you to gain a higher-level understanding or to get the gist of a situation. Dr. Uta Frith, the British AS researcher mentioned earlier in Chapter One, coined the phrase "central coherence" to describe this activity of the mind. NTs have a very strong drive to organize their experiences this way, or to use Dr. Frith's language, NTs have a strong drive for central coherence. In NTs, this drive for central coherence is present very early in life. There is research that infants as young as three months process input from multiple channels such as sight, hearing, and memory (for faces) in inclusive ways in their reactions to situations. If, for example, the mother of a three-month-old baby leans over his crib, calls his name, smiles, and reaches out her arms, the baby will smile back and begin to kick his arms and legs vigorously, expecting to be picked up. The infant has taken in information from multiple channels, understands the situation, and is able to anticipate what his mother's behavior will be. The drive for central coherence is fundamental to the NT way of thinking and plays a large role in the way we relate to others and navigate our world.

To summarize, NTs have a strong drive for central coherence. They take in relevant information from many sources and put it together to find a higher level of meaning. They use multisensory channels such as vision, smell, and sound. NTs pay attention to information such as where, why, and when the situation is occurring. They also register internal data such as feelings, memories, and knowledge that they have accumulated that is relevant to the situation. Because of the NT's strong drive for central coherence, the NT will put all of these kinds of data together in order to grasp the gist of the situation. Most of the time, especially if the situation is familiar except for some details, the NT will not even be aware that he or she is doing it; it happens automatically. If you question NTs about how they figured out the big picture concerning a situation, the usual response is, "I just know it." Let's look at what the strong drive for central coherence looks like in real life. Josh's story is a good picture of how this drive operates.

———————————————

Josh had met a very pretty college sophomore at the Mexican resort where he was spending his spring break. Josh was attracted to Jenny and wanted very much to go out with her. Jenny seemed to have her pick of the guys that were always hanging around her. Josh decided that if he wanted to start a relationship, he'd better figure out some special way to get her attention and to please her.

Josh, thinking about his goal of a date with Jenny, noticed that Jenny, a fair-skinned, red-haired girl, was very careful not to get sunburned. When she was out in the sun, she always sat under an umbrella and was diligent about putting on suntan lotion. Josh had also watched her when she was talking to her friends and noticed how her eyes would light up when she talked about her major, marine biology, and the marine animals she wanted to study. Thinking about what he knew about Jenny and what might be something special to do for a date, Josh remembered a folder he had seen in the lobby for an excursion in a glass-bottomed boat to see the marine life along the coast. Lucky for him he thought, the boat had a roof.

Josh saw Jenny later that day in the lobby. "Hey, Jenny, how'd you like to go out in a glass-bottomed boat? The tour guide said we'd see some pretty interesting stuff!"

"I don't know," Jenny replied. "I get sunburned awfully easily."

"No problem," Josh said. "The boat has a roof. When the boat brings us back, there is a pool there where we can swim with dolphins."

"Yeah, wow, it sounds like fun," Jenny said.

Josh's attempt to get a date was successful. He had taken in relevant information from many sources in making his decision about what to do. He had watched Jenny's behavior of staying out of the sun, he had listened to what she said about her interest in marine biology and sea animals, he had noticed her excitement (her emotions) about that subject, and he remembered the brochure about the glass-bottomed boat he had seen in the lobby.

Josh, a true NT, took in multichannel information (watching, listening, and monitoring Jenny's emotions). He called up his memory of the brochure for the glass-bottomed boat that he had seen earlier in the lobby (remembered information) and recognized that Jenny was very popular by seeing how the other guys were always around her. He needed to think of something that would be special to get her attention (past experience). Keeping all those things in mind, Josh, with his strong drive for central coherence, was able to figure out successfully how to get a date with Jenny.

Individuals with AS Have a Weak Drive for Central Coherence
Adults with AS seem to mostly approach the world detail by detail. They take in information one channel at a time (if they are listening to someone, they probably won't look at them). Dr. Frith has called this AS disposition to focus on detail weak central coherence. Dr. Frith and her colleagues believe the difference in the drive to central coherence, which is strong in NTs and weak in people with AS, may be the fundamental difference between people with AS and NTs. These differences in thinking style may be the result of or at least be related to the differences in brain structure and functioning between people with AS and

ANIMALS IN TRANSLATION

In her book with Catherine Johnson, *Animals in Translation,* Dr. Temple Grandin describes her experience when she was first learning about the cattle-processing plants where she consults. Dr. Grandin writes that in order for her to understand how the processing plant worked, she had to start by memorizing the smallest details of the process. It was only after a great deal of time spent studying details that she was finally able to see the process as a whole. Dr. Grandin described the details as suddenly just coming together one day.

NTs that is being found by researchers. New technology that allows us to see the brain functioning suggests that NTs and people with AS process information differently and in different areas of the brain. You can read more about differences in brain functioning in Chapter Five.

It is helpful to understand how these different cognitive styles play out in real life. When we look at Josh's story above, we can see that his drive to strong central coherence led him to take relevant information from many sources. He used that information to get a higher level of meaning—an understanding of what Jenny would like. Josh's way of thinking is a good example of the cognitive process of NTs and demonstrates how the NT cognitive style, the strong drive to central coherence, can be very useful in solving certain kinds of problems, especially if they are of a social nature. Don's story, below, will help us get some idea of how people with AS think and how a weak central coherence can be useful in different circumstances.

Don is a librarian at a liberal arts college. He graduated from the college several years ago and has worked there ever since. His school years, including college, had been very stressful. His AS made it difficult for him to relate to peers, and he often felt that he didn't fit in or that other students didn't offer to include him when they were doing things together. But things were better most of the time now. He liked his work and the predictability of his life. The people with whom he worked respected his careful attention to detail and his wide-ranging knowledge of facts.

A very successful alumna had recently left the college a large sum of money for a new library, and Don was asked to join the team that was helping to plan the new building. Don, who is not very comfortable with people, was a little reluctant to join the team, but his supervisor insisted that he could be helpful. The planning team was working with the architect who was designing the building, and the members of the planning team were being asked for their input about what they thought the new library should be like.

On the day it was Don's turn to give input about what he thought would be important in the new library, he showed up with a number of computer printouts. The printouts contained detailed records for the last four years that documented the changes in the way the library was being used by the patrons. Over that period of time, the number of people doing research by going online in the library had increased by 400%, whereas the number of those seeking help to use the reference books section of the library had dropped by half. The planning group was surprised by the data. Although the planning team recognized that there were more people going online, no one thought the change to online research was that dramatic. As a result of Don's detailed data and analysis, the new library will focus on computer access rather than book stacks. As a result, it will better serve the student population.

Don has a preference for detail and enjoys collecting facts. He is interested in computers and was very skilled at using them; students knew that and often came to Don for help. Don kept a record of the times he helped students, and he became interested in how many students were using computers instead of books. He decided to find out by also keeping track of how many students came to the reference book section when he was working in the library. He became engrossed in tracking this information, which he loaded into his computer. When Don was asked to join the planning team, it was easy for him to analyze his information and present it to the planning committee.

Don's carefully documented data showing the student shift from books to computers was very valuable to the planning group. Because it was actual data instead of opinion, less time was spent arguing different positions that were based just on what people "felt," and it was easier for the planning committee to come to a decision. Don's attention to detail and his love for information in the form of facts are good examples of the AS preferred way of thinking. Don has weak central coherence and was not interested in a larger context. He had collected the information because it interested him. Don was not thinking about the big picture—that the library might be constructing a new building—so his results were not contaminated by any personal agenda. Don's weak central coherence was useful because, in this case, it meant his data collection was objective.

When AS-NT Cognitive Styles Cause Problems

The stories of Josh and Don highlight the value of the two cognitive styles: the NT strong drive to central coherence and the AS weak central coherence. In Josh's case, his strong drive to central coherence made it possible for him to get the gist of a complicated social situation and led to him figuring out a way to be successful in getting Jenny's attention. Don, with his focus on details, had gathered facts about the way the library was being used. These data gave clear information about the way the library was actually being used and how the new building should be designed. But Don was not thinking about how the information could be used when he was collecting it. It was only when his supervisor insisted that he be on the planning committee that a use for Don's information became obvious. Dr. Frith and her colleagues think that one of the vulnerabilities of AS is not that a person with AS does not have information, but that he or she does not see the relevance of the information to the problem at hand.

We've seen how the two cognitive styles of weak and strong central coherence can be effective in certain circumstances. But what happens when an adult with AS and a person who is NT, with their different cognitive styles of weak versus strong central coherence, have to deal with a situation together?

Phyllis and her adult daughter Bernie are getting ready to go to a family wedding. Phyllis is excited about seeing her niece get married and doesn't want to be late. She wants to give Bernie, who has AS, advance notice about when they are leaving since Bernie is more comfortable if she knows what is going to happen.

"Bernie, get ready. It's time to go," she called as she went upstairs to get her purse and car keys. When Phyllis came back down the steps, Bernie was nowhere to be seen. Phyllis began calling to her and searching the house. Finally, in frustration, she wrote a note to Bernie saying she was going to the wedding by herself because she couldn't find her.

Phyllis hurried out to get into her car, which was parked in the driveway. Much to her surprise, Bernie was sitting in the car. Phyllis asked, "Where have you been? I've been looking all over the house for you. We're going to be late!"

Bernie responded, "You said it was time to go. So I got into the car."

Phyllis felt frustrated and angry. It's hard for her to keep in mind that Bernie doesn't think the way she does. Bernie gets focused on a detail in a very literal way and doesn't think about the bigger picture. When she heard, "It's time to go," she left and got in the car. Phyllis felt very frustrated by Bernie's behavior. Bernie couldn't understand why her mother was mad at her when she had just done what made sense.

DIFFERENCES IN AS-NT DRIVES FOR CENTRAL COHERENCE

NT—Strong Drive	AS—Weak Drive
• Multichannel input	• Single-channel input
• Prefer gist or big picture	• Prefers detail, accuracy
• Good memory for gist	• Good memory for facts
• Sees things as part of a context	• Sees things independent of context

The cognitive differences between NTs who have a strong drive for central coherence and people with AS who have weak central coherence very often result in both parties being frustrated, angry, or upset. Understanding that the differences are not based on thoughtlessness or a lack of consideration, which is how they are frequently experienced, but that they are the result of neurological differences, helps both individuals with AS and NTs to feel less distressed when the disconnects between them happen. They no longer take things personally.

Executive Function and AS

To meet our goal of learning more about AS-NT cognitive differences, we need to understand other ways in which the cognitive styles of individuals with AS differ from those of NTs. An important difference involves the ability known as executive function. Executive function is the ability to organize activities to complete tasks efficiently, or to put it differently, to plan and carry out the steps necessary to complete a task or behavior. It is also the ability that lets us learn from experience and not get stuck doing things that are counterproductive, such as spending time playing computer games when you are supposed to be at the computer to write a work report.

We know that executive function comes easily to NTs, whereas individuals with AS tend to have problems with it. Executive function is based on a number of mental abilities. To start with, it requires cognitive flexibility, which is the ability to consider different possible responses. Executive function also requires the ability to identify what is relevant and to be able to not act on ideas that are not useful or important in this particular situation. Executive function requires that you be able to learn from experience and to adjust your behavior based on feedback from the situation. It means you must remember the rules about what is appropriate and what is not and make the right decision for the event. Executive function means that you are able to keep your goal in mind at all times and that you are able to identify each step needed to achieve it. Individuals with AS tend to have problems with a number of the skills required for executive function and, especially when they are young, are likely to have serious problems organizing their activities and getting things done in an efficient way. To the extent that people with AS are impaired in their capacity for executive function, they will have difficulty managing their lives.

Cognitive skills required for executive function
- Having cognitive flexibility
- Recognizing what is relevant to the situation
- Learning from experience
- Holding in mind and using rules appropriate to the situation
- Holding a goal in mind at all times
- Identifying and executing each step needed to reach a goal

AS and the Lack of Flexibility
A key skill in effective executive function is the capacity to be cognitively flexible. NTs are able to consider many alternatives, but individuals with AS find it difficult to be flexible. Once individuals with AS have focused on something, it is hard for them

to consider anything else. This is true whether it concerns just thinking of different ideas or something more critical. People with AS tell us that once they begin thinking about something or become involved with something (especially if it interests them), it is difficult, sometimes impossible, for them to shift attention and think about or do something else. This problem may involve something as simple as looking at a flower or something that has broad consequences for the entire family.

Eleanor is married and has two young teenagers. She works as a chemist for a pharmaceutical company. She went on a sailboat for the first time while on a business outing that she was required to attend. She became obsessed with sailing and decided to spend her annual bonus on a sailboat. Eleanor took sailing lessons and soon began spending a great deal of money on equipment for the boat. Eleanor, who has AS, insisted that her husband and children accompany on her sailing outings on weekends and vacations. At first, her family enjoyed the sailing, but as time passed, her husband and children wanted to spend their free time doing things that reflected their own interests. When they refused to go sailing with Eleanor, she became angry or withdrew and would not interact with her family. The stress in the house became unbearable, and her husband insisted that the couple seek counseling. Eleanor could see nothing wrong with her behavior and insisted that her family needed to become more expert at sailing. In her mind, that would solve the problem. Her husband and children began to pull away from her, and the children viewed her behavior as very selfish. It was difficult for Eleanor's family to understand that the intense focus on the sailing was part of her AS, and Eleanor, because of her AS, could not let go of her need to sail at every opportunity.

The reason that it is so difficult for people with AS to shift focus, or "shift set" as it is often called, is not known. People with AS usually talk about the problem of not being able to shift set as if it is not under their control. They report that at times, even if they want to, they cannot stop what they are doing and get involved with something else. Whatever the cause of this lack of cognitive flexibility, it interferes with the executive function ability of a person with AS, since executive function requires that the individual be flexible and consider alternatives in his or her planning.

Learning from Experience

Learning from experience plays a major role in executive function. In executive function, there are two ways we use learning from experience. First, we use the feedback we get from the things we do in the present experience to learn what works and what doesn't. Second, we use things we have learned from previous relevant experiences. Learning from experience means that we understand what's going on in a situation and why what we did resulted in a certain outcome. We can then apply that learning to the new situation. To do this, we need to get the gist of situations and recognize the similarities of the situations. We know that to get the gist of something, we need a strong drive for central coherence. So, a strong drive for central coherence plays a major role in learning from experience. People with AS have difficulty getting the gist of the situation. What's more, they tend to take what they experience very literally. Any differences between the two situations, no matter how minor or unimportant, will likely get in the way of people with AS seeing the similarity of the situations, and they will not be able to transfer their learning.

Serge can't walk on his own because of his advanced Parkinson's disease. During his neurological assessment, it was also determined that he had AS and Tourettes syndrome. His adult children and their families live in other towns and are only able to visit occasionally. Serge has round-the-clock home health aides and visiting nurses to monitor his health needs. He's had problems getting along with some of the aides over the past year and has fired them. He's pleased with his new aide, Mary Sue, who now works for him five days a week. "I feel safe when Mary Sue is here," Serge told his family. Mary Sue frequently told Serge about her problems with finances. She was always behind on her bills but did not seem to worry about paying them.

Serge's family was shocked when a cable company's representative contacted Serge to collect a large and seriously overdue bill. Serge didn't have cable, but some investigation revealed that Mary Sue had used Serge's social security number (Serge had a good credit rating) to get cable service for herself and her family. "I need the cable so my kids have something to do when I'm here at work," Mary Sue told Serge. Mary Sue promised Serge that she would disconnect the service and pay the bill and that she was sorry for using his social security number without his permission.

Several months later, Serge received a phone call about a past due loan payment from a finance company. Once again, the loan was not Serge's. Mary Sue (who had a very bad credit rating) had again used Serge's social security number to get a loan from the finance company. Serge's family was upset. "You have got to let Mary Sue go." Serge refused, saying that, "Mary Sue is the only one I feel secure with. She told me that she took out the loan so her children could go to the dentist and that she will pay it back. I'm not going to fire her."

Several months after the loan incident, a collection agency for a new car company contacted Serge about payment on a large, expensive van. Serge denied having bought such a vehicle, but the collection agency replied, "We have your signature as cosigner on the auto loan." "I did not sign for a car loan. I've had my car for five years," Serge insisted. Serge's family contacted the local police, who began an investigation. Mary Sue had tricked Serge into signing the form for the auto loan by telling Serge that it was a form to prove that he employed Mary Sue. Mary Sue had told Serge that she needed the form to be able to rent a new house, so Serge had signed the form. It was only after the police brought fraud charges against Mary Sue that Serge accepted that she could not be trusted, and he fired her.

Serge did not put Mary Sue's behaviors together in a way that he could see that Mary Sue could not be trusted, no matter how nice she was. Serge didn't look at the big picture when Mary Sue used his social security number the first time, and so he failed to realize that she was not trustworthy. He did not see the pattern of Mary Sue's dishonesty the second time she had used his social security number and again had taken advantage of him. As a result, Serge refused to fire Mary Sue. Fortunately, when Mary Sue once again used Serge's social security number to buy the van, the police intervened and insisted that Serge fire Mary Sue.

Serge's story is an example of the difficulty some individuals with AS have in learning from experience. He did not learn from the cable problem that he could not trust Mary Sue, and he did not fire her. As a result, Mary Sue continued to take advantage of him twice more.

The Importance of Executive Function

We all use executive function in our daily lives. Many of the situations we face on a daily basis have become routine, and so executive function is less critical. We can better see how crucial the capacity for executive function is when we have to deal with new situations. When we are faced with a new problem to solve, we rely on executive function to help us cope with the situation. For example, if we are about to go skiing for the first time, we'll make a mental plan of what we need and how and where to get it. We'll get the information we need, whether it is by asking a friend who is a skier or researching skiing on the Internet. From past experience, we'll know that we have to make travel arrangements, and we will recall how we have done that other times. We'll know that it is appropriate to wear warm clothes, not swimwear, and so on. Using our ability for executive function makes it possible for us to successfully plan and take the skiing trip. Individuals with AS may be affected more by difficulty with executive function at certain stages of life when they face new kinds of challenges.

Midlife Problems with Executive Function
A substantial number of psychiatric referrals of people in their fifties that involve marital or other adjustment problems often involve AS and problems with executive function. In a very few cases, AS has already been diagnosed; in others, it becomes apparent when working with the individual. This is a period of life when there are often many sources of stress—career stress as the AS individual reaches job levels where there is an increased demand for people skills, the requirement for more emotional intimacy as the children leave home, or the recognition by individuals that they are not likely to advance beyond where they are now. For people with AS, any or all of these situations that demand they solve new, often complicated problems may result in their having a failure of executive function. Because the person with AS is not able to solve the problem, serious difficulties may result that lead one or both partners to seek counseling, as the couple can no longer cope.

Summing It All Up
This chapter has focused on differences in the cognitive or thinking style of people with AS and of NTs. Individuals with AS show a strong preference for detail, whereas NTs usually look for the gist or higher-level meaning of situations. Dr. Uta Frith has called this difference in cognitive style the drive for

central coherence. She suggests that this difference in cognitive style—a strong drive for central coherence in NTs and weak central coherence in individuals with AS—may be the fundamental difference in the way NTs and people with AS relate to the world and one of the sources of misunderstandings between the two. The drive for central coherence is a very useful concept when trying to understand the many disconnects that happen between NTs and people with AS. It helps to explain how differently the two groups read situations and react to situations. We've looked at the strengths and vulnerabilities in both strong and weak drives to central coherence and how the different styles work better in one situation versus another.

We've also looked at how people with AS tend to have problems with generalizing learning and difficulty with executive function. These problems can cause issues between individuals with AS and NTs; what's more, the nature of the problems usually confuse NTs because they don't understand that people with AS think differently. "How can someone who seems so smart and so capable in many ways have so much trouble dealing with life?" is a question we often hear in the consulting room. The behavior may be seen as deliberate, selfish, or otherwise negative. By understanding that the problems in functioning the person is having result from he or she having AS, and by having an understanding of the nature of AS, it's possible to identify the types of things that might cause problems and act to prevent them. The outcome for both the NT and the person with AS can become more positive, and it gets easier for the person with AS and the NT to bridge the two cultures.

CHAPTER FOUR

Understanding Others:
The Theory of Mind

"I told you that I didn't want Joe to step foot on any of our property ever again. You promised me that you wouldn't bring him here. I thought we had an agreement. That was Wednesday morning. Weren't you paying attention? I can't believe that you did this!" Barbara was clearly upset and angry as she looked at her husband, who was sitting next to her in the office.

Dan replied rather woodenly, "But Joe wasn't on the property. I needed him to help me move that equipment in our barn. You know I can't move it alone. I drove right up to the barn and opened the door. He stepped out right into our barn. He was never on the property. I did keep the agreement." Barbara responded, "I understood that what we had agreed to was that Joe would only work with you in your practice not do things here at our place."

The disagreement between Dan, who has AS, and Barbara, who is NT, concerned an employee, Joe. Joe works part-time in Dan's business. Recently, Barbara found Joe in their house twice, although he had no reason to be there. Joe explained that he had come in to use the bathroom, but later Barbara found that there was money taken from her purse. The second time she found Joe in her house, all the change was gone from a jar on the bedroom dresser. No one else had been in their house during that time, and Barbara was sure that Joe had taken the money. She was quite upset and a little uneasy with the idea of finding herself alone in the house with Joe; she just didn't trust him. Dan agreed with her that Joe had taken the money. Barbara wanted Dan to fire Joe, but Dan refused. He thought he wouldn't be able to find anyone else who would work as well as Joe did with the large animals that he cared for in his veterinary practice. Barbara was uneasy with Joe and didn't trust him. But she knew that Dan worked very hard and put in long hours in his practice. She also knew it was not easy to find employees willing to do manual labor in the area were they lived. Barbara suspected that it would probably take a lot of time to find someone to replace Joe, if they even could. She wanted to come up with a solution that would work for both her and Dan. After thinking about it for a while, Barbara suggested to Dan that he could continue to use Joe to help with his practice but that under no circumstances was Joe to ever step foot on their property. Dan was satisfied and agreed to the arrangement. The incident in the barn on their property had happened several days after they had made the agreement. Both Barbara and Dan felt that they had right on their side.

Dan picked up his baseball hat and began to twirl it between his hands. After a moment he said, "I don't know what you want from me. I didn't let Joe on the property. I did what you said. All you do is criticize me. You think I never do anything right." Barbara started to answer, but then shook her head. "It's always like this," she said. "It's like we live in two different worlds."

Barbara was more right than she realized. She and Dan have come up against a fundamental difference in the way they think and relate. Barbara, being NT, has a theory of mind. Dan, having Asperger Syndrome (AS), has "mind blindness." In many ways, they are in two different worlds. In the world of interpersonal relationships, the two ways of being are "worlds apart."

Theory of Mind and AS-NT Cognitive Differences

What does theory of mind mean? Theory of mind is the term used to describe the innate capacity of NTs to know and understand that other people have thoughts, feelings, and desires that are different from their own. When we say innate, we mean that NTs are probably born with this ability. We know that even very young children realize that others have a mind of their own and that they may think, feel, or want different things from what the child wants. NTs, from childhood, automatically pick up on nonverbal cues in social situations that allow them to understand other peoples' state of mind. Nonverbal cues are things such as posture, tone of voice, direction of glance, and other subtle indicators in which NTs engage to indicate what they are thinking and feeling. We'll be talking more about nonverbal communication later.

100

ROLE PLAY

We all have minds. Our mind holds the knowledge, be-
liefs, and desires that make us who we are. As young
children grow, their minds develop and they begin to be
aware of who they are and that there are others around
them. Their play begins to include taking on the role of
others, such as Mommy or Daddy. If we watch this role
play, it's clear that when a child is playing that he is
Daddy, he is imitating his father and the way his father
thinks. He will have a dialogue with his teddy bear as
though he, the child, is the father and the bear is the
child. The child will make up a scene, such as scolding
the bear for doing something wrong. Or he may tell the
bear goodbye and that he has to leave for work now, but
that he will play with the bear when he comes home.

It's clear from observing the child playing that he is
assuming the role of his father, and the things the child
says make it clear that he is aware of how his father
thinks. The child recreates his father's thinking and can
imagine new situations and figure out how his father
would probably react. This type of play, which usually
begins around age four, clearly indicates that the child
realizes his father has a mind of his own. The child has
a theory of mind.

Young children with AS may role play, but the quality of this role play is different. It's an exact reproduction of activities or roles they have seen. The play usually has a script or routine that the child does not allow to be varied. The child's play has a quality of mimicry rather than reflecting an understanding of the other person's mind.

It's different for people with AS. They don't automatically understand that others have their own thoughts and feelings and that these other people may want something different from what the person with AS wants. In fact, many people with AS don't seem to be aware that others have minds of their own. Because of this, Simon Baron-Cohen, a Cambridge University–based AS researcher, has coined the term "mind blind." Mind blindness means that you do not understand that others have a mind, which is the case for many people with AS. In their behaviors, their interactions with others, and their thinking, people with AS do not take into account the thoughts, needs, and feelings of others. They focus on the situation from only their own perspective. In other words, individuals with AS tend to be blind to the internal life of others.

What Can We Learn from Dan and Barbara's Story?
The episode that happened between Dan and Barbara gives us some insight into what can happen when someone with AS,

who is "mind blind," and an NT, who has a theory of mind, try to discuss a problem—especially one that involves emotion. When Barbara was thinking about the problem with Joe, besides taking into account her own feelings, she included thoughts about Dan that were based on her theory of his mind. Dan did not say to her, "I work very hard." He didn't mention that he was worried about finding someone else with Joe's ability to work with animals. Barbara was putting herself in Dan's place and thinking about the way she thought he would be thinking. Using her theory of mind ability, Barbara took into account what she thought Dan's wishes and needs were and tried to come up with an agreement that took both her and Dan's wishes and needs into account.

Because of his AS, when Dan thinks about the situation, he's almost certainly not going to take into account what is in Barbara's mind if she has not specifically told him. In fact, it's not likely that he would be aware that she was thinking her own thoughts and has her own needs. His thinking is based on the details of the situation and his focus is on the facts. Unlike Barbara, Dan does not try to put himself in Barbara's place and take into account what she might be thinking. Dan relies on the facts from his perception and logic to see if a solution meets his needs.

In clinical work, we are told repeatedly by NTs who have AS spouses that they can't understand or predict their spouse's behavior. They say they are never sure what their spouse will do next, and sometimes it makes them "feel crazy." From Barbara's perspective, she couldn't believe that Dan had brought Joe back on their property after they had made their agreement. Dan's behavior seemed to Barbara as though he was deliberately using her exact words to get around his promise about Joe. It felt disrespectful and as though he was playing games with her. In situations like this, it is as though NTs are blind to the minds of the individuals with AS. They simply cannot believe that the person with AS didn't understand the agreement the way the NT did. And people with AS get frustrated because, from their perspective, they believe that they have kept their word and that NTs should say exactly what they mean. It is a fundamental truth that both people with AS and people who are NT can be blind to the mind of the other. Bridging these two cultures is a huge task indeed.

A Lack of Awareness

Many of the problems between Dan and Barbara occur because this couple has no awareness that they each think in very different ways. When Barbara talks to Dan, she assumes that he has a theory of mind and that he will automatically put himself in her place and think about her needs, feelings, and wishes. As a result, Barbara assumes that Dan will take her thoughts and feelings into account in his thinking and his behavior. It never occurred to her to tell Dan the chain of thought that resulted in the agreement they made about Joe. Barbara is an NT, and in the NT culture, it is taken for granted that others have a theory of mind and will understand what is meant, even if it is not stated. When Dan doesn't take Barbara's feelings and needs into account, she doesn't know that it is because he has AS. She feels that he doesn't care about her or selfishly just wants to do what he wants. She ends up being hurt and angry.

Dan's mind operates in an AS style. His thinking focuses on details, and Dan doesn't usually see the needs of others. Because Dan lacks a theory of mind, or has a much underdeveloped one, it doesn't even occur to him to try to put himself in Barbara's shoes and to try to understand what is in her mind. As a result, Dan doesn't understand that Barbara has needs and wishes that are different from his own and alter his behavior accordingly. He will do what he thinks is the logical thing, based on what he understood the agreement to be, and will feel misjudged or criticized if Barbara is unhappy with him for what he has done.

Rules to Avoid a Misunderstanding

Better understanding between people with AS and NTs means that both parties must be aware of the differences in the way NTs and people with AS usually think and relate. There are two good rules to follow to help avoid this kind of misunderstanding:

1. If you are an NT, don't make any assumptions that the person with AS will automatically put themselves in your place and understand your needs. Be sure to say exactly what you want and why you want it that way.

2. If you have AS, recognize that there is a lot of information that is in an NT's mind that you might not be aware of and that for the NT is pertinent to the situation. Ask NTs exactly what they mean or want and why it is important to them.

This is a good place to emphasize again the importance of a diagnosis for someone with AS. The diagnosis alerts us to the fact that these differences in thinking style and understanding exist and that we must be prepared to deal with them. After all, looking at how complex these differences in thinking style are, without some guidepost, none of us are likely to stumble into understanding these complicated interactions!

One of the values of knowing a diagnosis is that it provides a framework for looking at misunderstandings when they occur in a rational instead of an emotional way. If we know that people with AS and people who are NT tend to think very differently, the misunderstandings become a problem to solve not an emotional offense. Barbara interpreted Dan's behavior as an indication that he didn't care about her feelings of fear and her desire to feel safe. Barbara hadn't told Dan those things but instead assumed that he would put himself in her place (theory of mind) and understand her feelings.

Dan responded to Barbara's statement that he didn't keep his promise with anger, because he thought that he had kept his promise. He had taken what Barbara said in a literal way, and did not let Joe step on their land. As a result, he felt she was criticizing him unfairly. The truth about the situation was that it was a clash of the AS-NT cultures. If Dan and Barbara are to live together with less distress, they will need to understand the ways in which they are different and take these into account when they are dealing with one another. Remember, Barbara will need to say exactly what she means, and Dan will need to check to make sure what he is hearing is what Barbara really wants.

AS-NT Communication and Nonverbal Communication

Many people with AS do not register the nonverbal cues that NTs use to express their feelings, thoughts, and wishes and that other NTs automatically read and take into account. Nonverbal communication is information that NTs convey through posture, tone of voice, facial expression, etc. Dan had listened carefully to the words that Barbara had said when they were making the agreement about Joe, and he had made his promise based on the words she said. Dan was careful to keep those words in mind when he brought Joe to the property. From his way of thinking, Dan had kept his promise. What Dan didn't know was that Barbara's words were a kind of code for a great deal of information and meaning. Much of Barbara's meaning was conveyed through tone of voice and facial expression. When Barbara said she didn't want Joe "to step foot on any part of our property," she was communicating in a nonverbal way, through the emphasis in her tone of voice, how strongly she felt about keeping Joe away. People with AS don't tend to understand this kind of nonverbal communication. Nonverbal communication doesn't even register with many people with AS, or if they detect a change in voice or facial expression, they likely will not be able to interpret it. Not only was Dan "blind" to Barbara's mind, but he heard only the spoken words of her communication. Dan did not know that he had missed a large part of what Barbara was conveying. Dan heard her words but did not know that there was much information that Barbara was sending nonverbally. Barbara had assumed that he would understand her nonverbal communication and know exactly what she meant.

Some experts estimate that as much as 90 percent of human communication is nonverbal. It's easy to see why so many communication disconnects happen between people with AS (who tend to not recognize or understand nonverbal communication) and NTs (who depend a great deal on nonverbal communication to get their point across). One woman with AS described her problem of interpreting NT nonverbal communication as like having dyslexia. She had learned to watch for changes in NTs' facial expressions and could recognize voice tone changes, but she could not make sense of them, similar to how individuals with dyslexia can see letters but cannot decipher them into words. Those with AS often ask, "Why don't NTs just say what they mean?" It's a good question!

There are two kinds of problems individuals with AS may experience in dealing with nonverbal communication: expressive and receptive. Expressive nonverbal communication is when we engage in behaviors to communicate, such as a big smile to indicate we are happy to see someone. Receptive communication is our ability to register and interpret nonverbal communication. Both seem to be a problem for many people with AS.

Many individuals with AS have difficulty with expressive nonverbal communication, and this is easily seen. Other people, when they see the person with AS who has trouble with expressive nonverbal communication, will see the person as being stiff, a bit odd, or different. On the other hand, receptive nonverbal communication, meaning not registering or not being able to interpret others' nonverbal communication (like we saw in Dan), is invisible. Because of that, it can be much more confusing to individuals around the person with AS. We can see the outcome of the lack of interpretation, which usually looks unfeeling or callous, but we don't know what to attribute it to other than rudeness or malice on the part of the person who engaged in the behavior.

Theory of Mind and Nonverbal Communication

The relationship between a lack of a theory of mind and the inability to decipher nonverbal communication is not yet fully understood. It seems likely that they are related; if people with AS are not aware that others have minds that are different from their own, it is possible that there would be no reason to look for information that is not verbalized. As a result, the skill in interpreting nonverbal communication would not develop in people with AS.

Researchers are trying to piece together the puzzle of problems with nonverbal communication in people with AS. Research coming out of Yale reports some interesting findings that relate to differences between what people with AS and NTs look at when they are watching a film clip. The clip involves people in an emotionally charged conversation. The researchers, by tracking the eye movement of their subjects, can determine what the watcher is focusing on at any given point in time. They found that NTs watch the faces of the people in the film and pay special attention to the area around their eyes. The NT subjects also tend to look first at the person speaking, then shift focus to the person listening, as if watching for the listener's response. People with AS focus more narrowly, looking at the mouth of the speaker. This more narrow focus likely means that the person with AS misses changes in facial expression. Because we learn much of our behavior from watching others, missing these facial expressions because of their focus primarily on the mouth may mean that individuals with AS fail to learn and develop their own facial expressions.

Nonverbal Communication Over the Lifespan

People involved with individuals who have AS have noticed that as individuals with AS gain life experience, many begin to get an understanding of theory of mind and nonverbal communication. Research with new technologies suggests that when people with AS do demonstrate a theory of mind, the ability seems to reside in a different part of the brain than it does in NTs, or at least is processed in a different place. The capacity to understand theory of mind and nonverbal communication in people with AS also seems to be very vulnerable to failure when the person with AS is stressed or in an emotionally charged situation. It has also been observed that for many with AS, even though they may understand the concept of theory of mind intellectually, they are not able to use it in interactions with other people. The same is true for nonverbal communication. They may have an understanding of the concept of nonverbal communication, but are unable to decode it when they see it.

Empathy in AS

Ken loves repairing old appliances, and he's good at getting them back into working order. His family and others know that, and so they bring most of their things that stop working to him.

As a result, Ken and Janet's house is cluttered with broken appliances. The backyard and now the front porch of his and Janet's home are overflowing with old TVs and useless washers and dryers.

"Ken, you have got to stop taking in any more old appliances. I'm tired of the mess, and our neighbors are complaining. It's going to be a problem. I'm afraid they are going to go to the town to complain. Please get rid of some of these things!" Janet, Ken's wife, is so upset she is crying. She and Ken have had this conversation many times before. Janet is tired of living in a mess. The inside of their house looks like a repair shop. There is disassembled equipment and parts everywhere. Ken insists that Janet not move anything because he knows exactly where everything is, and he can easily find the part he needs. Janet long ago gave up inviting her friends over. There is no decent place to sit, and the dining room table is covered with old TVs. Janet is feeling more and more isolated and lonely. Ken spends all his time working on the machines and has no interest in doing anything with Janet.

Their neighbors are annoyed at the mess outside, and Janet is embarrassed when she happens to see them, although she tries to avoid them when she can. Ken's standard response to Janet's concerns is, "It's my house. I pay the mortgage. I can do what I want in it." Janet knows that once Ken gets started on a certain path, it seems to be impossible for him to change direction. Janet had told Ken many, many times that if he didn't get rid of most of the broken equipment he had around the house and let her clean up the place, she would have no choice but to leave him. Ken never registered that his wife was becoming more and more upset by the situation. He was completely surprised when she told him one Saturday morning that she was leaving and getting a divorce.

Ken never anticipated Janet's leaving him. Janet had told him many times that she was unhappy and embarrassed about all the junk. She had said over and over that she was lonely and didn't want to live the way they were living any longer. Janet's feelings did not register with Ken. Ken, who has AS, has difficulty with empathy. Empathy is the ability to be aware of the thoughts and feelings of others and to adapt our responses to take them into account.

In Ken's thinking, it was his property. He paid the mortgage. Ken didn't see the equipment as junk. They were machines that he could restore to working order, and his ability to focus on detail and think logically made him very good at it. Ken really likes being able to figure out how something should work and fixing it if it is broken. The information that the neighbors were annoyed and that Janet was embarrassed, frustrated, and angry weren't a part of Ken's picture of the situation. Because of Ken's AS, he did not feel empathy and, as a result, he was not able to understand Janet's or his neighbors' feelings.

Experiencing empathy depends on having a well-developed theory of mind. Ken's theory of mind is poorly developed, and he can't empathize with others. Not understanding Janet's feelings, Ken did not adjust his behavior to take into account her needs. If Ken had done that, it would have made Janet feel better about their marriage, and she might have been willing to stay. Because of his AS, Ken was not tuned in to Janet; he really didn't understand her and what she needed or thought. As a result, he was puzzled and very surprised when Janet left and got a divorce.

In Janet's thinking, she could no longer tolerate Ken ignoring her feelings. She loves Ken; he is kind and loyal. Being an NT, she cannot understand why he behaves the way he does. Janet doesn't understand that Ken's lack of empathy is because of his AS. After trying unsuccessfully many times to get Ken to understand how upset she was and how important it was to her for him to take her feelings and concerns into account, Janet decided her only option was to end the marriage.

Empathic Response and the Wish to Share Attention

People with AS not only have problems with feeling empathy but also often lack empathic response. Empathic response is the wish to share attention with others. This desire seems to be inherent in most humans. We can see a capacity for empathic response in very young children. They behave in ways that show us that they have a wish to get others to pay attention when something interests them and are interested in what others are interested in. Even before she can talk, when an infant sees her caretaker looking at something, she will look at the object, too. When the child is a little older, she will point a finger at an object she wants her parent to notice. The child will then look at the parent to make sure the parent is looking at the object.

As adults, we show an empathic response when we express interest in something that is of interest to someone else. A good example of this would be when two friends are together and one mentions to the other that she has recently seen an interesting television program. When her friend asks what the show was about, she is demonstrating an empathic response.

In Chapter One, we talked about Dr. Simon Baron-Cohen, an AS expert from Cambridge, and his interesting theory that AS is just an extreme form of the natural continuum of behavior rather than a disability. In a recent book, Dr. Baron-Cohen suggests that the human brain may be naturally wired toward one of two tendencies; one tendency is toward empathy, while the second tendency is toward systems and how things work. It has been a very provocative theory because Dr. Baron-Cohen suggests that females are more disposed toward being "wired" for empathy, whereas males are wired to be disposed to systematizing or determining how things work. While there are many people who do not agree with looking at gender this way, it is always useful to come across any ideas that may spur further research and better understanding of AS-NT differences and their cause.

Difficulties with Empathy and Issues Around Feelings
Difficulties with empathy do not necessarily translate into a lack of ability to have feelings. In fact, many parents of children with AS take exception to the idea that people with AS are cold or uncaring. These parents report that their children can be warm and affectionate with people with whom they are close (for example, parents or grandparents). These parents also say that despite known problems with empathy in individuals on the autistic spectrum, their children can often pick up feelings in these same

people to whom they are close, although the children do not always interpret the feelings correctly. A number of parents of children with AS believe that it's not that their child doesn't experience feelings but that the child experiences them too intensely and can easily become overwhelmed and confused by these feelings.

Summing It All Up

We have spent a lot of time looking at cognitive differences between people with AS and people who are NT. Our intent has been to try to look at differences in cognitive skills very carefully, one skill at a time. Obviously, cognitive processes usually involve more than one skill being used at any given point in time, so to look at them one at a time is somewhat artificial. We've taken this approach to try to help make clear the differences in the ways in which NTs and individuals with AS function. We've tried to demonstrate the impact of these different cognitive styles by providing clinical vignettes that illustrate them. We hope that reading about actual incidents between NTs and individuals with AS will help you understand how these differences play out in real life. In our clinical experience, it can take a long time to really gain an understanding of these differences and to be able to easily recognize them for what they are—expressions of the different ways of thinking by NTs and people with AS.

From working with adults with AS and people who share lives with them, we've found the most powerful tool we can give them is an understanding of how, to use Dr. Atwood's term, the two cultures differ. Dr. Attwood, you may remember, is the AS expert from Australia who writes and lectures extensively about AS. Understanding and accepting that there are very real differences provides a place to begin to improve communication and interaction between the two cultures. It allows us to focus on rational problem-solving, not reacting with anger or frustration.

Recognizing, or even gaining an understanding of, the AS-NT differences doesn't mean the differences won't still frustrate and annoy. Most likely, both individuals with AS and NTs will continue to wish the other person would change or that he or she was different. We need to acknowledge that neither NTs nor people with AS will change very much, probably in large part because the differences appear to be hardwired. What understanding can do is to help us better anticipate the situations that are likely to go wrong and help us to solve the problems, hopefully less emotionally, when upset does happen. But unless we understand these differences, we will continue to be mind blind to one another.

CHAPTER FIVE

Understanding AS and Its Impact on the Brain

Y‌ou know, Ted, you're doing a good job of learning how to dance!" Elisa smiled at her husband.

Ted responded, "You know I never had a chance to try to dance when I was in high school or even college. If they were dancing somewhere and I was there, I'd just sit in a corner and watch. I always felt left out," said Ted.

"That must have been kind of tough," said Elisa.

"Yeah. My sister was always my champion when I was growing up; she was always on my side. So I asked her to teach me to dance. She said okay, and we would practice in the family room. Then one day when I wanted to practice, she said, 'No, not anymore.'"

"Why didn't she want to practice with you anymore?" asked Elisa.

Ted continued, "Well, she said she hated to tell me, but that I have two left feet, which at first sounded weird, but she said it meant that I was not well coordinated, which is true. I know that. Then she said, 'And, boy, you ain't got no rhythm!' Then we both started laughing."

"What was so funny?" asked Elisa.

"Well, when we practiced dancing, I kept getting out of step and banging into her. Sometimes it was frustrating, but she didn't get mad, so we usually ended up laughing."

Elisa had met Ted at a friend's wedding, where he had hung around watching her dance. But he had puzzled her; he had never asked her to dance that night even though she was expecting him to. Elisa understood the reason later, when after they had started dating, Ted told her he didn't know how to dance and asked her if she would teach him. Remembering this, and thinking about her own experience teaching Ted to dance, Elisa thought, "His sister is right on both counts. He does have two left feet and he sure doesn't have much of a sense of rhythm." She felt a little sad for Ted and would have liked to hug him to let him know how much she loved him and that she understood how important learning to dance was to him. But she knew that Ted did not like being touched unless he initiated it. His skin was so sensitive that he couldn't wear starched shirts, and when he bought new clothes, he always complained about how uncomfortable they were until they had been washed many times.

Elisa thought about what Ted said about his sister being his champion. She hoped that Ted felt that way about her; she loved him a great deal, but there were many things about Ted that were "different" and that often confused her. Not only did he have trouble getting into the rhythm of dancing together, Elisa couldn't get their steps to match when they walked together. And although Ted was super smart, sometimes he just didn't "get things." He didn't seem to see the big picture, and he wouldn't understand when she talked to him about what a situation meant. Being able to focus was one of Ted's real strengths, though. When Ted decided he wanted to do something, he was completely focused and even had trouble thinking of anything else. He wanted very much to learn to dance and had insisted on practicing dancing almost every evening since they got married. Sometimes she almost thought that the reason Ted married her was that she was a good dancer and could teach him. Yes, there was no question that when Ted made up his mind to do something, he was going to do it. Ted's boss, when Elisa had met him, had told her that he had never known anyone who got so focused on what they were doing as Ted did, and he often gave Ted the most complex technical problems because Ted wouldn't give up until he had solved them. And with all their practice, Ted had finally learned to dance.

Symptoms that Result from Differences in the AS Brain

Ted has Asperger Syndrome (AS), and he sometimes struggles with the symptoms. He is hypersensitive to touch and some textures, and certain sounds "drive him nuts." He is extremely bright, and because he has the ability to focus on anything that interests him, he has been very successful at most things he decides he wants to do. This focus has a downside, however, because it is hard for him to shift his attention to anything else when he is absorbed in what he is doing. It is difficult for Ted to understand nonverbal communication, and he has difficulty understanding other people (lack of theory of mind). And quite often, Elisa playfully reminds Ted that he has a one-track mind that gets so lost in the details that he doesn't see the big picture (weak central coherence).

Understanding AS and its strengths and vulnerabilities is a challenging task. It's not obvious how the wide range of symptoms, from trouble with communication and not understanding others' state of mind to hypersensitivity and various sensory and motor problems, fit together. Making the picture even more complicated is the fact that many people with AS have extraordinary capabilities in some areas, such as, for example, having remarkable memories for facts or being able to do complex mathematical problems in their heads. All told, it is a very mystifying picture. What we do know, however, is the brains of people with AS operate differently, and some of the structures within the brain seem to be different than those of NTs. (We will be talking more about that later.) Learning more about the nature of these differences in the brain will help us get a better understanding of the fundamental nature of AS. The purpose of this chapter is to provide some basic understanding of the impact of AS on the brain and the symptoms that probably result from these AS-related brain differences.

Problems with Understanding Research Findings:
Dealing with Inconsistent Diagnoses

The DSM-IV-R (*Diagnostic and Statistical Manual of Mental Disorders: Fourth Edition*) began officially recognizing Asperger Syndrome in 1994, and although autism research has garnered a lot of support and attention, it has only been recently that AS specifically triggered research. Despite the fact that research is now being conducted on AS and its impact on the brain, there are still problems because there is a lack of agreement about the criteria that must be met to diagnose AS. Scientists who review the research done to date on AS report that the criteria used to select the AS subjects for participation in the research are not always clear. As a result, it is hard to compare the various studies.

However, the need to understand the whole spectrum of autistic disorders has led to the establishment of autism spectrum disorders research centers of excellence at a number of universities. There are now efforts underway, especially in those settings, to carefully define the criteria for AS that will be used to identify research subjects for the AS research now being conducted. These centers are proving to be fertile grounds for advancing our understanding of AS and the other pervasive developmental disorders.

New Technologies Are Providing
New Ways to Understand the Brain

Technologies such as functional magnetic resonance imaging (fMRI) have made it possible to see the brain working and have allowed researchers to broaden their focus from the structure of the brain to also look at the way it works. The fMRI allows researchers to identify areas of brain activity by tracking an increase in blood flow to the active area. This capacity allows researchers to compare activity in the brains of people with AS with activity in the brains of NT control subjects.

Theory of Underconnectivity:
A Critical Brain Difference in AS versus NT Brains

Several neuroscience researchers have been finding evidence that a fundamental difference between AS versus NT brains is the degree of "connectivity" between divisions of the brain. For example, a recent finding by Dr. Marcel Just and his team at Carnegie Mellon Center for Cognitive Brain Imaging has generated a lot of interest in the community studying AS. Using a brain-scanning technology that identifies areas of brain activity by measuring blood flow, the research approach focuses on looking at how the brain works not on how it is built. Studying AS males with IQs that are in the normal or higher than normal range and NT control subjects, the neuroscientists looked at brain activity while the research subjects solved tasks that required several areas of the brain to work together. The researchers found that, in the AS group, the network of areas involved in the task were less synchronized and that an integrating area of the brain was less active compared with the NT control group. Dr. Just proposed that brain deficiencies in coordination and integration may be the fundamental problem in AS and the other autism spectrum disorders. Coordination and integration are terms that refer to the way the brain works.

The human brain has different centers that could be compared to computers and that are responsible for certain kinds of activities, such as speech or processing input from our senses, like smell or taste. These centers are specialized, and there are circuits in the brain that connect these centers. We might think of these circuits as cables that connect the computers (the various specialized centers). The brain functions by communicating in a synchronized way between the "computing" centers and coordinating the information coming from these centers. The brain then puts the collected information together (integration) in a way that lets us understand and act on our experience. The brains of people with AS and the other autism spectrum disorders don't seem to work together in a cooperative way. The coordination and integration process just described is necessary to solve complex problems that require a number of specialized areas to work together to reach a solution. High-level thinking, or put another way, solving problems that require information from many of the specialized areas of the brain, is often impaired in AS and the autism spectrum disorders. Researchers refer to this problem of poor coordination and poor integration as "lack of connectivity" or "underconnectivity" and theorize that the autism spectrum disorders, which include AS, are brain-wide disorders that limit the coordination and integration among brain areas.

A Possible Explanation for AS Special Abilities
This theory might help to explain one of the mysteries of AS and the other autism spectrum disorders—the fact that some

individuals on the autism spectrum, including individuals with AS, have normal or even very superior skills in some areas (the output of individual specialized brain areas as defined above; these special skills are often referred to as "islets of abilities"). At the same time, many other types of thinking (that require input from a number of brain areas) are impaired (such as social communication). If, as Dr. Just and others hypothesize, the problem in AS and all of the autism spectrum disorders is underconnectivity (or the inability to connect the various specialized areas of the brain and to put that information together in a meaningful way), the brain might compensate for the problems in communication between the different specialized areas by enhancing the specialized centers themselves. This could lead to unusual skills in one brain area, such as the ability to do rapid arithmetical calculations. Highly developed skills such as this are frequently seen in individuals with AS and the other autism spectrum disorders. The fact that the specialized area develops relatively independently of the other specialized brain centers may result in that center becoming "expert" in that particular function—a common finding in AS.

Differences in White Matter: A "Cabling Problem"?

Dr. Just's and his colleagues' findings primarily involve white matter, which functions as the "cabling" to connect the various grey matter areas of the brain that do the computing when we are problem-solving. The findings of white matter abnormalities dovetail with research findings of other autism spectrum disorder investigators, who have also found abnormalities in AS brain white matter. Because we know that complex thinking and problem-solving require coordination and integration of input from many brain areas, anything that would interfere with communication and integration would make it difficult for the AS brain to solve broad intellectual problems or to be able to interpret complex social interactions, two areas of function impaired in all the autism spectrum disorders.

The theory of underconnectivity is still being researched, but it is very consistent with Dr. Uta Frith's theory of weak central coherence in autism spectrum disorders, discussed in Chapter Three. The research finding of insufficient connectivity and poor integration between different brain areas suggests that the weak central coherence noted in AS has a biological basis. The lack of connectivity and problems with integration would probably interfere with the AS brain coordinating and integrating the different kinds of information (as described in Chapter Three) necessary to get the gist of a situation.

Sensory Problems and Movement Disorders Linked to the Cerebellum

The cerebellum is the lower back part of the brain. It is responsible for regulating balance and the movements of limbs as well as playing a role in speech and sensory modulation. All are areas of function that are frequently disturbed in AS and autism spectrum disorders. Dr. Eric Courchesne, a neuroscientist from the University of California, San Diego, demonstrated (and it has been validated by other researchers) that specific areas of the cerebellum are abnormal in AS and the other autism spectrum disorders and that, in at least certain cases, the cerebellum is smaller in AS brains than in NT brains. These research findings of differences in the cerebellum of the brains of people who have AS would help to explain the sensory problems and movement disorders that were noted in Ted's story.

What Causes Autism Spectrum Disorders?
No one is sure what causes AS and the other autism spectrum disorders, although there is a general agreement that genetics plays a definite role. Research indicates that there are probably several genes involved, but it is likely that, in some cases, other factors play a role as well. For example, in identical twins (who have the same genetic makeup), if one twin is diagnosed with autism, the second twin only has a 60% likelihood of having the diagnosis;

PHYSIOTHERAPY

Understanding that AS-related difficulties are the result of physiological differences offers some hope that remedial activities such as physiotherapy may improve some of the problems mentioned above. Physiotherapy is a health care profession that uses various physical approaches such as exercise to promote and maintain physical, psychological, and social well-being.

this suggests that environmental factors likely play a role. There is a good deal of research underway to identify what the other factors might be, but no conclusions have been reached so far.

Hope for Early Diagnosis

In Chapter Two, we talked about the importance of being able to make a diagnosis early in the child's life so that interventions can begin as soon as possible. Work by Dr. Courchesne on brain growth rate differences in AS may lead to the ability to diagnose the condition by using head circumference measurements in the first years of life. Basically, Dr. Couchesne's findings are that the rate of brain growth in AS and the autism spectrum disorders during the young child's development differs from that of NTs.

A Pervasive Developmental Difference in People with AS

In Chapter Two, we noted that AS is part of a group of disorders called the pervasive developmental disorders. The pervasive developmental disorders are so called because their effects involve a number of functions, such as hypersensitivity to sound, problems with motor coordination, and the inability to read nonverbal cues. All of these functions involve the brain and the way it works and are common difficulties seen in AS. Neuroscientists are beginning to identify the differences in the structure and functioning of the AS brain, which may be responsible for these problems, as discussed above in the sections on underconnectivity and cerebellum research. The exact way in which the brain and these problems are linked is not yet understood, but there is agreement in the AS research community that these factors are most likely linked in some way. But until we have a clear picture of just how brain differences translate into the problems of AS, it's important to address the impact of the problems on the individual with AS and the issue of how these problems may be misinterpreted by NTs, often in a negative way.

Developing a Better Understanding of AS-Related Difficulties

The specific set of difficulties experienced may differ from one person to another, but any or all of the difficulties associated with AS may cause problems in interacting with other people. If it's not recognized that the difficulties are all a part of AS and its impact on the way the brain functions, others may find the behaviors annoying, rude, or selfish. Recognizing the kinds of symptoms associated with AS brain differences will help individuals with AS and NTs be more accepting of these differences and learn to cope with them. Let's look at some of these possible problems.

Sensory and Auditory Integration
What Is Sensory Integration?

Our senses work together. Each sense works with the other senses to put together in our minds a complete picture of who we are physically, where we are, and what is going on around us. Sensory integration is the critical function of the brain that is responsible for putting this composite picture together so that we may understand who we are, where we are, and what is happening around us.

Problems with Sensory Integration

Individuals with AS may have very hypersensitive reactions to many kinds of sensory stimulation such as touch, sound, smell, taste, and visual stimulation. A teenage girl with AS couldn't tolerate being on the beach, although she longed to be part of the group that went there. Her sensory hypersensitivity made the movement of the waves and the sparkling light on the sand and water overwhelming, and she would experience intense panic. Because of this symptom, she was limited in the things she could do; this in turn affected her social life negatively. Talking and thinking about her problem was upsetting to her. She said her hypersensitivity made her feel defective, and her friends thought that she was "weird" because of her problem. Ted, in the opening story of this chapter, did not like to be touched. This issue could be serious in a marriage, because a partner needs to express and receive affection. The list of possible sensory problems in AS is a long one and can affect individuals around the person with AS. An NT woman who was a gourmet cook felt frustrated because her husband, who has AS, could not tolerate the sound of the kitchen exhaust fan but complained that the smell of garlic cooking made him feel nauseous.

These sensory problems are real and can be very painful and stressful for people with AS; they are not "being picky" as one parent of an adult with AS described it. The discomfort the person with AS experiences goes well beyond "not liking it." It can literally be unbearable.

WHAT CAN BE DONE ABOUT PROBLEMS WITH SENSORY INTEGRATION?

If you have AS:

1. Note and write down the kinds of sensory problems you have as you experience them. Share this record with people who are close to you and let them know that these kinds of things are difficult or impossible for you to manage because of your AS. Experiment with different ways to manage your sensory problems. If, for example, your skin is extremely sensitive to certain textures, such as wool, look for clothing that is made from some other kind of textile, such as cotton.

2. Try to avoid situations where you can't control sensory input. If you can't avoid such a situation, and it is reaching the unbearable point, let someone know you are not feeling well and leave.

If you know someone with AS:

1. Recognize and understand that these problems are real for individuals with AS. Remember how you hated the scratch of fingernails on a chalkboard? Magnify it a thousand times.

2. If you need to do something (for example, cook the garlic), warn the person with AS, or schedule the cooking for when he or she is not around.

What Is Auditory Integration?

Auditory integration is the ability of the brain to hear information and to process it in such a way that it is meaningful. People with AS and other autism spectrum disorders typically have problems processing auditory information. Listed below are several forms of auditory integration problems.

Problems with Auditory Integration

Auditory integration problems can take several forms.

• The person with AS may not be able to follow spoken directions that include more than two points.

• The person with AS may have difficulty hearing you speak when there are other competing sounds such as voices or any kind of distraction.

• The person with AS may have auditory sensitivity that can be to certain kinds of sounds and pitches, regardless of how soft or loud.

• The person may be able to hear speech sounds but is not able to understand the meaning of the sounds. A related form of auditory integration problem is not being able to distinguish between certain sounds, for example B versus P. As a result, the person with AS may not be able to comprehend what is being said.

Problems with sensory and auditory integration can make life more difficult for people with AS, and it may be hard for the people around them to not become impatient with these problems. People with AS may speak too loudly or too softly; they

೧ೡ

WHAT CAN BE DONE ABOUT
AUDITORY INTEGRATION PROBLEMS?

If you have AS:

1. If you are getting directions that involve more than two points (such as a grocery list or directions to an office building), carry a small notebook or 3 x 5 index cards and jot down the information.

2. If you are in a situation where there is too much competing noise or distraction, you are better off explaining the problem and trying to move the conversation to a quieter, less active spot.

3. There are some training methods for people with auditory integration problems. These are listed on the Autism Society of America Web site.

Go to www.autism-society.org for more information.

If you know someone with AS:

1. Don't assume the person with AS wasn't listening if he or she has difficulty following directions. It is hard for many individuals with AS to follow and remember a long list of items or instructions. You'll have more success if you write out the instructions for the person with AS.

2. Understand that the odd pattern of sensitivity to sound is just that. The fact that your college-age son can listen to ear-splittingly loud rock music doesn't mean that his inability to tolerate your beloved little dog's yipping isn't real. AS can be a merciless master, and the kinds of problems the person with AS experience don't always look logical!

may need help to recognize this. They may have a strong preference for a certain kind of fabric or not be able to tolerate a clothing label touching anyplace on their body. This may seem to the NTs around them that the AS individuals are just complaining. Again, these problems are real and are most likely the result of the way the AS brain is wired. It's important to be aware that these sensory problems may become much more severe when the person with AS is especially tired or stressed. NTs can help by understanding that the person with AS does not have control of these problems and by trying to cooperate as the person makes an effort to cope.

How Some AS Adults Manage Sensory Problems
Adults with AS have usually figured out ways that work for them to manage sensory problems. One man with AS had trained himself to be able to fall asleep almost instantly in situations where he was at risk for sensory overload as his way of coping. It became easier for his wife and family when they found out that he was not doing this to be rude but that it was a part of his AS.

A young woman with AS had learned that if she told others she was feeling ill, she was able to escape from many settings that overstressed her (the stress did indeed make her feel ill). She was a member of a college choral group that traveled by bus to other campuses to give performances. Although she wanted very much to participate, she would invariably have to be "rescued" with a flight ticket home to escape being overwhelmed by all the sights, sounds, and scents of a group of 20 young women crowded onto a bus. Her parents became less impatient with this behavior when they understood that it was a result of her AS.

Motor Coordination Difficulties

Most people with AS have at least some motor skill deficits. The problem may be gross motor coordination, like Ted's dancing ability in the story above, or it may be fine motor skill difficulties. (Computer word processing is a true gift to many people with AS who struggle with the fine motor skills required for handwriting.) We've already mentioned the often-unusual gait of people with AS in Chapter Two. Ted also had problems with spatial judgment that led to his bumping into his dancing partner.

These motor and coordination problems may make it hard for someone with AS to participate in a team sport, but others may be excellent athletes in individual sports such as bicycle racing or swimming. Choosing an activity that does not involve having to coordinate with others may lessen the stress that comes from not being able to participate in team activities.

Finally, for many individuals with AS, their single mindedness may help them develop a skill that they really want. Ted told

Elisa he had always wanted to be able to dance; he not only made sure to find a partner who could teach him, but he organized their lives so that he could practice and learn to do so.

Timing and Rhythm Problems
Timing
AS can affect certain individuals' ability to have a good sense of time or to be good at sequencing activities. Problems with sequencing activities means that it may be difficult for the person with AS to know where to begin a task that requires an orderly step-by-step approach involving more than two steps.

If you have AS and time or sequencing is a problem:
1. Make it a habit to always wear a watch and train yourself to be aware of it. One successful businessman with AS always used a timer on his watch that beeped. He used it not only as a reminder for appointments but to mark the hours and help him keep track of time.

2. For sequencing steps of a task, once again, notes in a notebook or on small 3 x 5 index cards can be a quick and ready reference. If it's some new project that involves more than two steps to complete, it may be a good idea to ask someone to help you sort it out.

When thinking about the impact AS can have on some people's sense of time, I remembered an incident involving "marking time" that made quite an impression on me. It's sometimes said that AS is the "engineers' disease," and indeed some studies of the families of people with AS have found a higher number of engineers in their family background than would be expected by chance. While it is in no way a statement about AS and engineers, this particular experience sure demonstrated to me that engineers are at the least very conscious of time!

Shortly after I began doing consulting work at a very well-known technical laboratory, I had my first real "dose" of the engineering bent of mind. Soon after I had begun there, I was asked to attend an all-day meeting that brought together several different laboratories. The meeting began at exactly 8:00 a.m., and the first presenter's talk was scheduled to be an hour long. At precisely 9:00 a.m., over 300 watches beeped almost simultaneously. I looked around the room and noted that the only person who seemed at all surprised by what had just happened was me. The watches belonging to the speaker and the group vice president holding the meeting had beeped as well! The timed beeps continued on the hour for the rest of the day, and I had watched as several of the men made minute adjustments to their watches. By noon, the room was full of beeping watches that were perfectly synchronized—there wasn't even one little "off-center beep" left. I looked at the numberless, mute Movado watch on my own wrist and wondered what I had gotten myself into. I know now, many years later. The years of working with those brilliant research scientists and engineers were some of the most fascinating of my life.

Difficulties with Matching Rhythm in AS

Some people with AS have absolutely no sense of rhythm while some have a simply superb sense of it, especially when doing something alone, such as playing drums. Social rhythm can be a different story, and many with AS describe difficulties with matching rhythm with others. This may show up when they are trying to match strides walking, or it may be most problematic in trying to "catch the rhythm" of social conversation. Temple Grandin has written that she will probably never figure out how to fit into the rhythm, or give-and-take, of NT verbal exchanges.

Summing It All Up

Neuroscience researchers are beginning to unravel some of the brain differences that underlie differences in functioning between individuals with AS and NTs. In some cases, for example, "underconnectivity," the neuroscience findings fit well with research findings from other disciplines—in this case, the cognitive psychology theory of the weak drive for central coherence. These dovetailing findings help give direction for critical future research.

This chapter has also looked at some of the difficulties people with AS experience with motor coordination, sensory and auditory integration, and problems with timing and rhythm. The cerebellum area of the brain is involved in most of these activities, and recent research findings indicate that there are differences between the cerebellum of the brains of people with AS and the brains of NTs, suggesting there is a physiological basis to these difficulties. The physical differences in the brains of people with AS seem to cause problems that are often judged unfavorably as bad or careless behavior. For example, poor handwriting might be seen as carelessness or sloppiness—character faults that the person with AS could overcome if he or she chose to. The fact that there is likely a physiological basis that may not be under the control of the person with AS explains these sensory and motor problems and helps all concerned see these issues in a different and more accepting light.

Understanding that the differences in the brain that result from having AS affect many areas of functioning helps both the person with AS and his or her significant others to work together to cope with these vulnerabilities and increases the shared understanding of the world of AS.

CHAPTER SIX

Dealing with Emotions in the AS World

"I'm very disappointed. I thought things would be different when we moved here and that I'd find some women in my neighborhood to be friends with." Maggie continued, "But it turns out the women in my neighborhood are just like the women were where we lived in Chicago."

I asked Maggie, "Can you tell me why you are disappointed in these women?"

She continued, "It's always the same. In the beginning, they are willing to talk about interesting things. They'll ask questions like, 'Where did you move from?' 'Why did you move?' They seem interested in my pottery collection and ask about the different pottery studios where I've worked. But that doesn't last long. Before very long, all they want to do is gossip about other people. They say mean things about others." Maggie said.

"Maggie, what sorts of things do they say that upset you?"

It took a while to get a clear picture of what Maggie was talking about. The women she was referring to were other mothers she had met in a parents' meeting at the neighborhood grade school her daughter attended. The women, who all lived in the same area of town, often talked about what was happening with the people in the neighborhood. A lot of the conversation focused on who was feeling what and why, and the women would often mention how they felt about the situations they were discussing.

"Can you remember an example to tell me?" I asked Maggie.

"Well, yesterday afternoon, I was out getting the mail and Susan, my next door neighbor, came outside. We said 'hello,' and then she asked me if I could pick up her daughter at school when I picked up mine. I said, 'Yes, I would.' Susan said the reason she couldn't pick up her daughter was that she had promised Cinde, another neighbor, that she would help her take her twins to the pediatrician. Cinde's husband Jim was supposed to help her, but he had to be out of town on an unexpected business trip. Then Susan said, 'It's terrible, don't you think, that Jim has to travel so much.'"

I was a bit puzzled at this point, because Maggie repeated the conversation as an example of how "mean" Susan could be. It took a lot of questions for me to finally understand that Maggie thought that Susan was criticizing Jim for traveling so often. Maggie thought Susan was being mean and unfair, since Jim's job required that he travel.

Despite my efforts to help Maggie see that Susan was really sympathizing with Cinde and Jim about the fact that Jim's work demanded so much travel, Maggie couldn't accept any way of looking at the situation except her own. She was sure that Susan was being critical of Jim.

"I don't want to be around mean people, so I avoid Susan. But the trouble is all the women in the neighborhood say mean things," Maggie finished.

————————————————

Maggie had come to therapy because she was unhappy. She and her husband Tom had moved to this town when her husband's company transferred him to a new job. Tom was very busy with his new position, and Maggie was on her own a lot. Maggie had trouble with change, and it was difficult for her to make new friends. She had gone through a very bad period in college when she didn't feel accepted or included and had been diagnosed at that time as having Asperger Syndrome (AS). Maggie's AS-related difficulties were playing a role in her having trouble adjusting to the move. Not only did Maggie have to learn about how to get around in a new area, she had to adjust to many changes in their routine. Tom had to work a lot of hours in his new job, and Maggie felt lonely. She had hoped that she would be able to make some friends in the new town. But, because of her AS, this was proving to be difficult. It is hard for people with AS to understand the minds and emotions of others. Because she has trouble understanding emotions, Maggie felt very uncomfortable in dealing with them—even hearing about emotional feelings in conversation. She could see no point in talking about people and their feelings. She consistently misread it as criticism when someone talked about their feelings about what was happening in other people's lives. Maggie had learned a lot from her therapy when she was in college. But there are still many things about NTs that are hard for her to understand. Emotions, and NTs' interest in them, are on that list.

AS and Difficulty Managing Emotions

It used to be that many people who worked with autism spectrum disorders tended to feel that people on the spectrum were cold and did not experience emotion. We now know better. Individuals with autism spectrum disorders, including those with AS, can and do have very strong emotions. The problem however is that many people with AS lack emotional competence; they have trouble recognizing and understanding their own feelings as well as the feelings of the people around them.

What Is Emotional Competence?

"Emotional competence" is a term used in the mental health field to describe an individual's ability to understand and effectively manage feelings or emotions. You have emotional competence if you can recognize and identify your feelings and are able to understand them, cope with them, and use them in an adaptive way. It's a pretty tall order, but it's a challenge we are all faced with all the time, and even very young children are expected to develop skills in this area.

Recognizing Our Feelings and Managing Them Successfully

When we recognize the emotional response that we have to someone like the annoying driver described at right, we do it by

EMOTIONAL COMPETENCE:
AN EXAMPLE OF MANAGING NEGATIVE FEELINGS

You're driving on a narrow local street that has a fair amount of traffic going in both directions. Suddenly a driver passes the car behind you, cutting in very quickly behind you. The driver of the car begins tailgating you and flashing his lights. There is a car in front of you— you have nowhere else to go, and suddenly you realize you are very angry at the driver's behavior. The thought crosses your mind that you'd like to jam on your brakes to indicate your anger at his bad behavior, but fortunately at the same time that idea crosses your mind, you are also aware that it would be a foolish and dangerous thing to do. You might cause an accident— or with all the reported cases of road rage, you might even get shot! Your only option is to get away from the driver and his obnoxious behavior. You look for the next turnoff and leave the road. By the time you drive around the block to get back on the road, the annoying driver is no longer in sight. You pull out into traffic and get to your destination safe and sound. Your emotional competence has kept you from making a potentially serious mistake.

becoming aware of our internal experience. In this case, the internal experience is unpleasant and makes us feel as though we want to strike back at the person causing us grief. The feeling is accompanied by physical signs and symptoms. We're breathing a bit faster, our heart rate may be a little increased, and our hands are locked tight on the steering wheel. We can feel our response becoming more intense, and the wish to strike back is getting stronger. At the same time, a part of our brain recognizes that if we do strike out, we'll get in trouble. By identifying the feeling as anger, recognizing that it is growing in intensity, and using our common sense (good judgment based on what we know or have experienced), we deliberately begin to "turn down" the anger and realize that it will be better if we get away from this situation with the driver who is provoking us. Now that we are aware that we are angry and that the bad driver is the source of our anger, we decide to get off the road at the next exit. Our judgment has told us that getting away from the situation is our best option, since we can't change the annoying driver's behavior. This emotional competence protects us from being overwhelmed by our feeling of anger and, as a result, making a potentially dangerous response. Emotional competence lets us manage our lives with less risk and a lot more effectiveness.

Maintaining Emotional Competence Over the Lifespan
Emotional competence is a skill we have to hone all our lives. Each stage of life brings new challenges, and we've got to work through those challenges to find ways to cope effectively. As young children, we had to learn to wait for summer and school vacation. It was tough to deal with the feelings of impatience,

but there was no way to speed up time, so most of us, instead of dwelling on the wish for vacation to begin, focused on other things like playing games with friends. For many of us, getting to high school meant that someone we were attracted to might not be attracted to us; we had to learn to manage our feelings of disappointment and focus on feelings of hope—to be willing to look for someone else to care about. Marriage, and the long-awaited joy of the birth of a first child, brings us happiness, but we also find out that the birth of a child brings fatigue, annoyance, and frustration because of the seemingly never-ending interruptions in sleep. We can't nor would we want to walk away from our child, so we have to figure out new ways to cope with the feelings we are having.

Developing Skills for More Complex Situations

In many new situations, an old way of coping, like getting away from the annoyance (which we discussed in the driver scenario) may not be suitable. When we have a child, for example, he or she is our responsibility, and we've got to figure out how to manage the ambivalent feelings that we are experiencing. It may be as simple as reminding ourselves of how much we love the child and that the baby will soon be able to sleep through the night. Still another option might be discussing our feelings with the baby's other parent and enlisting some help to share caring for the baby in the middle of the night. Both of these options mean we have learned to handle our emotions in new ways that are better suited to the new situation.

Generalizing Learning:
Applying Emotional Competence to New Situations

As NTs gain experience over time, they generalize what they have learned about being emotionally competent and learn to adapt existing skill at emotional competence to new situations. Their responses become more complex and sophisticated. For example, we might find ourselves annoyed at a neighbor and feel that we would like to completely ignore her. But, we know we will probably be living next door to one another for many years to come, and to ignore her would probably be awkward. We may also know that she is president of the parent-teacher association at the school our child attends and that to offend her might have negative consequences for our child (for example, if she complained about us to one of our child's teachers). So, instead of ignoring her, we decide that the best way to deal with her is to be nice but keep our distance and have as little to do with her as possible while still being polite. This decision is a good example of more highly developed emotional competence. But, every once in a while, we find ourselves stymied in dealing with our emotions in a particular situation; suppose, for example, if we feel very angry, but we are not able to get away or to change anything about the situation that is making us angry. This means our newer, more sophisticated strategies to manage emotions, the ones that we have learned over the years of gaining emotional competence, won't work for this situation since we have so little control. At such times, we may find ourselves resorting to tactics of managing our emotions that we learned when we were very young and that still prove to be very useful, such as, for example, counting to ten. When we can pick and choose what behavior we will engage in to manage our feelings, we are behaving flexibly. This flexibility to select any response (new or old) that will work effectively in a given situation is a form of emotional competence. Not too long ago, a friend laughingly told me about an interaction she had with the technical support staff for a computer company and how she had found herself falling back on an anger-management technique her grandmother had taught her when she was a little girl.

"For the first time, since I was probably eight years old, I had to count to ten, I was so mad! I was trying to get some help for a computer glitch and called the 800 number for tech support. The support center was not U.S.–based, and the technician obviously spoke English as a second language. The technician I was talking to must have been depending on a script to walk the user through a series of steps to identify the problem, starting with, 'Have you checked to make sure the computer is plugged in?' A reasonable question, no doubt, but I was in a hurry, and since I work with computers all the time, I had already run through all the standard checks. I was trying to hurry up the process and get him to listen to the problem I was having. What led to the 'count to ten' incident was the fact that each time I tried to hurry up the process by jumping ahead to my question, the man from tech support would go back to the top of the script and ask, 'Have you checked to make sure your computer is plugged in?'"

My friend had to have the help with her problem, so she had to stay on the line. She tried being polite and thanked him for his help but told him that she needed more sophisticated advice, a way she had learned to deal with people with whom she consulted at her job. But her tech support person wasn't prepared to deal with this move and kept reverting to his script. She realized after the second time or so that she had better just follow along with the script, or it would mean going back repeatedly to question number one: "Have you checked to make sure your computer is plugged in?" Casting about for a way to control her frustration so she wouldn't interrupt again and have him go back to question one, she found herself resorting to an old anger management tool—counting to ten under her breath.

Challenges People with AS Have in Expressing Emotion

Developing emotional competency is a challenge for many people with AS. They have difficulties in dealing with feelings, from identifying and understanding their own feelings and expressing them appropriately, to being able to recognize and adequately respond to the feelings of others. NTs often say that it is hard for them to be around someone with AS because many people with AS do not express emotions, either in words or through facial expression or body language. NTs will often describe someone with AS as "wooden" or "robot like." Because NTs rely heavily on nonverbal communication to understand others and use this information to judge how a situation is progressing (for example, "Are people interested in what I am saying? Is this meeting going on too long?

Did he understand what I said?"), this lack of nonverbal, or even verbal, emotional expression means the NT will have difficulty understanding what the person with AS is feeling or how the situation is going. As a result, without any way to capture this information, the NT will often feel uncomfortable or uneasy around a person with AS.

Bill, a senior manager in a technical organization, is donating blood to the blood drive his company is sponsoring. On the cot next to him is Ed, a computer expert in Bill's organization.

Bill exclaimed, "I'll be doggoned. Your blood is red just like the rest of us!"

"What do you mean? Of course it's red," Ed responds.

Bill continues, "I thought it would come out as a string of ones and zeros!" Bill, of course, was joking and referring to the ones and zeros of computer coding. Bill always feels uneasy around Ed because of Ed's expressionless face and monotone voice. Bill doesn't understand Ed, and since he is not comfortable being around him, he avoids him whenever possible. Because they had to spend the thirty minutes or so lying next to each other while donating blood, Bill resorted to his sense of humor as a way to hide his discomfort. Ed did not understand Bill; he thought Bill's remark about ones and zeroes didn't make sense. Ed has AS, and because his thinking tends to be very literal, he didn't get the metaphor, and so he didn't get the joke. Ed had no idea that it was his lack of expressed emotion, whether verbal or nonverbal, that made Bill uncomfortable. Ed didn't understand why Bill usually avoided him, but he did feel rejected by him.

The AS Preference for Facts Over
Feelings Means Losing Information

Some people with AS report that feelings are annoying, and they choose to ignore their emotions and insist on focusing on facts. One individual with AS was in a meeting where there had been some disagreement, which resulted in strong feelings. His conclusion was, "The world would be a better place if humans focused on facts, not feelings." There are probably a fair number of people, both with AS and NTs, who might agree with this sentiment (at least under certain circumstances), but if we step back and look at feelings, we can see that they are a very powerful source of information. Most of us don't tend to think specifically of our feelings as data, but our emotions play a very important role in our lives. For example, our feelings help us to form our identity. Ask a little girl to describe herself, and her first response is likely to be, "I am a good girl." Ask her what being a good girl means, and she's likely to say, "I do what my mommy and daddy ask me to do." If your next question is, "Why do you do that?" she will probably reply, "Because I love them and they love me" or "Because I want them to be happy."

So if we look at what the child has said, we can see that her loving relationship with her parents is at the core of how she sees herself or her identity. Emotions also help us to form our value system. When we do something for another person and experience a good feeling as a result, it reinforces caring behavior as part of our value system. The emotions of shame and guilt that follow bad behavior are so unpleasant that experiencing those feelings reduces the likelihood of our repeating the behavior and clarifies our value system from the perspective of things we do not do.

The AS Reliance on Strict Interpretation of Rules

Individuals with AS tend to be very rule-conscious and committed to following rules; in fact, children with AS often adopt the self-appointed role of rule enforcer, reporting rule infractions to teachers and in general policing what goes on in school or on the playground. It goes without saying that this makes them unpopular with other kids, and it's useful for parents to try to stop or curb this behavior. Individuals with AS most likely find rules helpful in making sense of their experience and as guidelines about what to do in what they often describe as the "unpredictable NT world." The shortcoming of depending on rules as a guidance system for our life is that there is no way enough rules can be written or that rules can be comprehensive enough to cover all situations. It is important to be able to use our judgment, which often includes our feelings about what is happening. If a police officer stops us for speeding, and we tell him we are on our way to the hospital where our husband has been taken for a heart attack, the rule says he should give us a ticket. But the officer, recognizing that the situation probably has us frightened, is likely to give a warning and let us go. We need feelings to interpret rules and recognize appropriate exceptions.

Research on Emotions and Judgment in Decision-Making

A new generation of scientists is studying the topic of emotion. For a long time, the common wisdom was that reason and emotion were in opposition and that emotion clouded logic and led to poor decision-making. The new research on emotion shows that emotion is integral to the process of good reasoning and successful decision-making. Dr. Antonio Damasio, a neuroscientist at the University of Iowa, and his colleagues studied a group of individuals who, because of neurological damage to specific sites in their brains, have lost the ability to experience certain kinds of emotions. These were people who, up until the time of the damage, had led very successful lives. After the damage that lead to their not being able to experience certain feelings, they are still completely able to reason and use logic, but many personal and social decisions are irrational and, more often than not, are poor life choices.

One of the most famous cases in the history of neurology involves a man named Phineas Gage, and his story is a both sad and fascinating one. Gage worked for the railroad in the late nineteenth century when the railroads were expanding westward. Gage's job was to set the charge and dynamite through rocky obstacles to create a level track for the rail bed. To do this, Gage drilled a hole in the rock and filled it with dynamite, tamping it down with a metal rod and, when the charge was in place, igniting the dynamite. One day, the charge went off by accident, driving the rod right through Gage's head. Gage was able to walk away from the accident, and in every way seemed intact, except in his ability to register his emotions.

Despite the fact that Gage did not appear to have suffered any serious damage and despite how intact his intellectual reasoning was, Gage lost his capacity for good judgment. He had a lot of difficulty managing his life and was seen by his friends as "not being Gage," an expression used to indicate that he was not the person they had known. Research many years later revealed that the area of Gage's brain that was damaged was an area that is important in awareness of emotional state. When Gage could no longer be aware of what he was feeling, he could no longer make good decisions about how to live his life.

It's important for people with AS to work on improving emotional competence, including recognizing and identifying their own feelings. It is possible, with some effort, to begin to understand your feelings and to learn to cope with them more effectively. There are some steps that will help improve the ability to recognize, manage, and use feelings more effectively.

How People with AS Can Improve Their Emotional Competence

- Decide it is important to understand and manage your emotions. Managing emotions is like getting physically fit. If you don't commit time and effort to doing it, it won't happen!

- Find someone you respect—someone whom you feel handles emotions well—and use that person as a role model. People with AS are exceptionally good at being able to pattern themselves after someone. Exploit this skill!

- When you are trying to learn to get in touch with your feelings, make it a point to stop—especially when you are interacting with someone you trust—and try to get in touch with what you are feeling. By asking people you are with what they are feeling, you may get a clue as to what your emotional state is. You may be reacting to the situation in the same way. Pay attention to the physical signs of emotion. Clenched fists usually mean anger; drooping shoulders are often a sign of sadness.

• Look around you at what is going on. Pay attention to try to see if there is a link between what is happening and what you are feeling.

• See if you can link the situation and feeling with a time you have experienced them together before. Keep a diary of these experiences; you'll likely remember your experiences better if you write them down. What's more, people with AS are often better at writing about their feelings than talking about them.

• Take some quiet time to think about how you have handled a situation that involved feelings and ask yourself if there is a better way you could have handled it. Write it down in your diary.

• Review your diary regularly to refresh your memory.

• Understand that it is harder to learn about something and understand it when you are upset or there is too much going on. Don't get discouraged; just try again when there is less pressure.

Difficulty with Recognizing and Talking About Feelings

Some people with AS lack the words for emotions, a condition called alexithymia. If you have AS and have trouble identifying

KEEPING A JOURNAL

Many people with AS, while they may have difficulty talking about feelings, write very eloquently about their emotions. Getting in the habit of keeping a journal of emotional experiences can be extremely helpful to people with AS in enhancing understanding of their emotional life and increasing their emotional competence.

emotions or naming them, it may be helpful to work with a friend and write down a list of the simplest emotions—happy, angry, and sad. Your partner or friend can help you find pictures that show these expressions clearly. Study and ask questions about what clues to look for in each emotional state. For example, are the corners of the mouth turned up? That usually means the person is happy. If the corners of the mouth are turned down, the person is likely sad. Using a mirror, practice making expressions with your face as a way to begin to have a sense of how to express feeling. (A note of caution: Get feedback from a friend, and be careful not to overdo the expression.) A quick and easy first step is to practice smiling back if someone smiles at you.

It's important to start with the simpler feelings. It can take a while to understand more complex feelings such as pride or embarrassment. It is also difficult to understand and be good at dealing with conflicting feelings. If a friend gets a promotion you wanted, it can be a struggle to identify that you have two feelings toward the friend—you like her, but now you also envy her. By the way, this is one of the more difficult tasks for people who have AS; they have a long history of seeing things as black or white—it can't be two things at the same time. Count it as a victory when you grasp that you are having both feelings!

Being Overwhelmed with Feelings

As we have seen a number of times, people with AS may have polar opposite experiences. Some may have trouble recognizing or even experiencing their feelings, while others may have such intense feelings that they become overwhelmed. What can people with AS do when they are feeling overwhelmed by emotion and are having trouble managing their feelings?

Three Ways a Person with AS Can Cope with Being Overwhelmed by Feelings

1. Practice relaxing by using deep breathing (yoga is a great way to learn this) or any relaxation technique. If you don't know relaxation techniques, search the Internet, or buy a book on relaxation exercises at a bookstore.

2. Do something you know calms you. One man I knew told me that when he was stressed, he played solitaire on the laptop computer he took with him everywhere. It was a bit surprising when he announced he had played more than 14,000 games, most of which he won!

3. Don't awfulize! Awfulizing means thinking about all the terrible things that could possibly happen and reacting as if they could all happen at once (even if some of them were mutually exclusive!). A good question to ask yourself to get awfulizing under control is, "Will I die from this?" If the answer is "no," then it really isn't awful!

Anxiety and Depression: Common Emotional States in AS

Anxiety is the most commonly reported feeling by people with AS. It is not surprising that people with AS experience chronic anxiety. For someone with AS, coping with the confusion of the NT world, frequent change, and the demands of life (such as work and school) can be and usually is stressful. Fears of not getting it right, or of not being able to cope, take their toll and create feelings of anxiety.

We mentioned in Chapter Two that it is also common for people with AS to experience depression. Feelings of failure, hopelessness, or helplessness lead to feelings of depression. The experience of rejection, which is not uncommon in AS (NTs often find it difficult to understand people with AS and may turn away), may result in anger, which can then become depression if it is turned inward. Other sources of depression for people with AS may come about as a result of the person with AS not being able to live up to his potential because of difficulty communicating or because of any of the other problems associated with AS. These negative emotions can take their toll on individuals with AS and may have negative health consequences.

Some Ways People with AS Can Manage the Effects of Negative Emotions

• There is a lot of medical evidence that the simple act of exercising regularly can help with negative emotions. Exercise should be a regular part of your life.

• Listening to your favorite music is a good way to relax and change your mood.

• Stay healthy. Investigate healthy diets, and watch your weight.

• If you find yourself becoming upset in a situation, excuse yourself by announcing that you need some time alone to get your thoughts together.

• Practice, practice, practice writing or keeping a journal! It will help you to sort out your thoughts and feelings.

• Simple tactics, such as counting to ten before responding or envisioning something calming, such as walking on a beach, can often keep the feelings from escalating and make it a little easier to maintain self-control.

Understanding and Dealing with Unusual Behavior

Sometimes if people with AS aren't sure what they are feeling or they don't have words for it, they may make a response that is inappropriate, such as laughing when someone gets hurt. If you have AS and this happens, it's very helpful, when you are feeling calm, to let the people around you know that these reactions are sometimes uncontrollable. This early warning will help keep the other party from overreacting or taking it personally, which could potentially damage the relationship. A behavior goal for occasions like this would be to simply say, "I'm sorry. I'm feeling very upset and anxious."

It is often hard for some people with AS to follow a long set of verbal instructions or any directions if they are anxious. The stress of the situation may lead to an inappropriate response such as anger or silliness. A good strategy for someone with AS to fall back on at this time is to simply quietly say, "Sorry, I'm not sure what you would like me to do." If it involves more than two things, write it down.

Understanding What It Means If Someone in Your Life Has AS
The most important thing you can do if someone in your life has AS is to acquaint yourself with the way AS affects the individual. Understanding emotions are very difficult for people with AS— not just their own emotions but the emotions of those around them. If you are with someone who has AS, and you become upset, or react in a highly emotional way to something he or she has done, your feelings will be contagious, and the person with AS is likely to immediately become upset, too. It will be harder for the AS individual to respond to you appropriately, and the situation may escalate out of control. If you can't get your own emotions under control, it's best to excuse yourself until you feel more in control. You can then pick up the conversation and state in a calm voice what has upset you and what behavior you want changed.

160

If you are upset in response to the person with AS not taking your feelings into account, or reading your emotional expression, understand that criticizing him or her for this will get you nowhere. There is every chance that he or she won't have any idea what you are talking about—remember the problems with theory of mind? Your best chance to keep things from escalating is to simply, slowly, and in a calm, quiet tone tell the person with AS what you want.

Cautions about Emotions and Inappropriate Behavior

"Many times, I am sure he tried to provoke me until I lost it," Liza said to the other women in therapy group. "It proved to him that I was the crazy one and that he was in control. Then gradually, I noticed that what he was looking for was to provoke any kind of emotional response in me. He seemed to be treating our relationship like he was a scientist studying emotions and emotional responses. It was like he was thinking, let me do this and see how she reacts. Then I noticed that at one point he started mimicking my emotional responses, sort of trying them on. He often looked weird because his responses were so obviously inappropriate to the situation, and he would 'parrot' my exact words. He didn't even seem connected to what he was saying; it was just like he was reading a script."

We've seen a number of times that some individuals with AS will deliberately provoke strong reactions (sadly always negative) in their NT partner to watch the partner's response. While this seems to be done as a kind of living laboratory or a "class in emotions," and doesn't seem maliciously motivated, this behavior is extremely destructive to the unwitting NT. Liza in the above story was so provoked that she finally lost it and lashed out. She was then left with the pain of fearing that she had been verbally abusive to her AS partner and the shame of having behaved badly and contrary to her nature.

We all have our limits, and it is not reasonable to expect an NT to have unlimited patience or to tolerate verbal attacks. Some of the behaviors of people with AS can be profoundly destructive, and if the diagnosis of AS has not yet been made, the behavior will likely leave the NT partner devastated and with no way of knowing what has really happened and with no means of protecting herself from another such episode. In some cases, the person with AS will use "the silent treatment," which is an extremely damaging and subtle form of emotional abuse.

When the person with AS uses emotional withdrawal as a form of punishment when the NT has done something that makes him unhappy and he refuses to talk (the silent treatment), the NT has no way of knowing what has gone wrong or how to repair the situation. If the person with AS has not been diagnosed as having AS, the NT has no way of knowing that her partner is prone (because of problems with understanding others) to misinterpret situations. The person with AS will not see his role in what has happened and will blame the NT partner. What's more, people with AS will often feel justified in treating a significant other any way they chose because of the way they interpret marriage. In my practice, I have had men with AS state that they expect their partners to love them unconditionally and to treat them with unconditional positive regard—saying that is what marriage means. This obviously unrealistic expectation does not seem to go both ways, however, and the partner with AS may feel free to attack his partner, sometimes even physically.

Individuals with AS quickly establish patterns of behavior, especially if it is something in which they are interested and want to learn more about, such as studying their partner's emotional reactions, or if it gives them more control over the other person, such as verbal abuse. **It is very important for the NT to put a stop to these physically or emotionally abusive behaviors immediately. AS is not an excuse for bad behavior, and no one has the right to experiment on or abuse a fellow human being.** The person with AS should be advised, firmly and clearly, as follows.

What to say to avoid active provoking: You are deliberately provoking me to try to make me get upset and angry. I will not tolerate this. You must stop at once and never do this again. If you want to ask me questions about feelings, you may do so. But do not ever again deliberately provoke me.

How to handle withdrawal as a form of abuse: If the behavior is withdrawal, it may prove much more difficult to manage, because the person with AS feels he or she has the moral high ground or hasn't done anything. This self-righteousness needs to be confronted quietly but firmly and addressed as follows: I know you think that you are not at fault because you are not saying anything. Refusing to talk to a partner is a form of emotional abuse. This is unacceptable behavior, and I will not tolerate it.

People with AS, like the rest of us, do best in an emotional setting where they feel accepted and secure; but this does not mean that people with AS can do anything they choose, regardless of how the behavior affects others. The right setting for good, lasting relationships is a balance between firmness and receptivity. What's more, if you are an NT, make sure you have lots of relationships in your life to keep the balance you need for emotional support and validation, since the nature of AS will make it difficult for your partner to do those things for you.

Tips for NTs in Dealing with AS Emotions

There are times when individuals with AS will be truly overwhelmed and unable to manage themselves. You may learn to recognize the behaviors when your AS person is overloaded or overwhelmed. This will differ from one person with AS to another, depending on his or her personality. It may be argumentativeness, anger, or freezing you out by deliberate withdrawal, or it may be all of the above at different times. It is often difficult to determine what external events may be upsetting, and it is very possible that your person with AS will not be able to identify these events, or if he or she does, talk to you about them. But if you are willing to watch closely, you'll learn to recognize the signs. Eventually, if you're teaming up to improve communications, you and the person with AS may be able to partner to identify the problems together.

Tips for an NT Dealing with Emotional Overload in a Person with AS

• Recognize when the person with AS is overwhelmed.
• Don't take it personally.
• Listen to what he or she has to say. Is there a point?
• Don't attribute everything to AS. Present your own values and limits.
• Insist that the heart is as important as the head. Feelings count!
• Don't forget that AS is not an excuse for bad behavior.

Summing It All Up

Emotion is part and parcel of being human; it gives life color and flavor, meaning and motivation. The whole area of emotion is difficult for people with AS, and their difficulties become problems and difficulties for those NTs who share a life with them.

Just to recap, individuals with AS usually have problems with recognizing, understanding, and coping with their own emotions. It's important to understand that, for people with AS, this often results in them feeling anger and frustration. But in fairness, they cannot take out those feelings on the people around them. Individuals with AS, because of problems with theory of mind, also have trouble recognizing and understanding the emotions of others; they are mind blind.

These problems with recognizing and understanding emotions will have an impact on both people with AS and the NTs with whom they interact. When someone with AS tries to relate to an NT, because people with AS are not always in touch with their own feelings, they may come across to the NT as cold and distant. NTs may pull back from the person with AS because they don't feel warmth or welcome. The person with AS then feels rejected, which can be painful. Unfortunately, because of their problems with recognizing and expressing their own feelings and their problems with being emotionally related to others, a number of people with AS have experienced a great deal of rejection in their lives. It may be this rejection that in part accounts for the AS tendency toward negativity—a trait many people with AS share.

In the case where people with AS, because they are not good at nonverbal communication, miss all kinds of emotional information that NTs assume they read, NTs are hurt and frustrated that they are not understood. Trying to work through all these problems in any relationship seems like a lot of effort, but most people want someone to share their life with and may be willing to make the effort. Trying to work through emotional problems in AS-NT relationships is very challenging and may not always be successful.

One of the most difficult problems for an NT in an AS-NT relationship is not being able to share feelings, especially joy, with the AS person in his or her life. We don't know why, but people with AS rarely, if ever, rejoice in others' success, and they are usually not interested in what others are doing. In general, they aren't inclined to share emotional reactions to life's grief and joys. Some individuals with AS eventually learn that it is important to try to do these things for their friends or partners and will make an effort to do so. It can be difficult, since it is not a natural response for them and it is often done in a highly formal way. It is very gratifying when they have made the effort, and it is usually a statement about how important the relationship is to them.

Individuals with AS often find having several relationships, such as being friends with other couples, draining, and sometimes the NT will gradually drop contacts with friends to accommodate the person with AS. But most NTs need relationships, and we urge the NT, whether a partner, parent, or friend, to make sure you keep lots of relationships in your own life to help you keep the balance you need for emotional support and validation.

Dr. Paul Ekman, a psychologist at the University of California, San Francisco, is one of the editors of *Emotions Inside Out: 130 Years After Darwin's Expression of the Emotions in Man and Animals.* Dr. Ekman, who has helped revive the field of the study of emotions, remarks that "expressing emotions is serious business." Dr. Ekman goes on to say "emotion is relevant to everything from counterterrorism to successful marriage." Putting a lot of work into developing and using emotional competence is a richly rewarding investment for people who hang in there and learn to do it. And the work of developing emotional competence is one more way to improve the contact between the AS and NT cultures.

CHAPTER SEVEN

Understanding the Personal Impact of AS

My work is to try to understand others and to work with them to clarify and solve problems they face. The problems come in all shapes, sizes, and importance. The person may be dealing with something that to others seems trivial and unimportant, like the woman who was very upset because she couldn't get the caterer she wanted for her daughter's wedding. Or the situation may involve working with parents who have just been told that there is nothing more the medical profession can do for their 14-year-old son who has bone cancer. Are the problems comparable? In a way, it doesn't matter—emotional/psychological pain is pain, and no one can know for sure what it is like for the individual experiencing it. My work with people with Asperger Syndrome (AS) has made it clear to me that their struggle to make sense of the world of NTs can be a very stressful, even painful, one. Even more importantly, because AS is the result of the differences in the way the AS brain is structured and functions (as discussed in Chapter Five), there is as yet no known way to alter those differences even if someone wanted to. As a result, the effort to compensate will be lifelong. By understanding the way AS effects functioning, it's possible to identify some solutions to make it easier for people with AS to cope with the NT world.

When I first began working with what I've come to think of as the world of AS, I was struck by how complicated it was to deal with this condition, for both the person with AS and for the people with whom he or she shares a life. The complications have to do in part with how pervasive the condition can be. It can affect many areas of the person's life. These problems include such things as the problems they often have in trying to read emotions and understanding other people, as well as sensory problems such as the serious discomfort they may experience when they hear certain sounds. This chapter will focus on a number of the experiences and challenges that people with AS have told us about or that have been written about previously. We'll also cover some ideas on how to handle these challenges.

Who Has AS?

There are two ways to answer this question. The first answer might be that probably one person has AS in every 250, so chances are we all know someone with AS. The second answer, and the more interesting one, is all kinds of people. AS is the condition not the person, and many argue that it is really not a condition but a variant of normal behavior. There is no AS personality, and people with AS come in all shapes and sizes and with as much variety in personality traits as the rest of the world. Some people with AS are extremely shy; others are more outgoing and love to be the center of attention. I've known people with AS who are self-proclaimed "geeks" who live for their computer "fix," or musicians who are so caught up in the world of music that there is little time for anything else in their lives. So there is no particular AS personality, but the presence of AS means that to some degree or another, individuals with AS relate differently than NTs do to the world and the people in it. This chapter will identify those differences from the perspective of the people with AS and also how that in turn affects the NTs who share lives with them.

The Impact of AS
We don't yet know why, but the degree of impact of AS varies widely, and some people have a "touch" of AS, while the degree to which others' lives are affected is much more severe, to the point where their lives are ruled by the condition. We also know that the nature of the impact of AS differs from individual to individual, and not everyone with AS will have all, or even the same, symptoms. The end result is that it is not possible to come up with one-size-fits-all solutions to managing AS. To try to make this discussion as useful as possible, we'll cover the spectrum of the kinds of issues associated with AS, even though not all will apply to all people with AS.

AS and the capacity for change

The very nature of AS makes it difficult for the person to identify problems and change his or her behavior. Here are some of the reasons:

- AS often interferes with the ability to predict the impact of one's actions on someone else. AS causes problems in understanding others' minds. AS causes difficulties reading nonverbal communication.

- AS often causes rigidity in thinking or behavior. Once a position has been taken or a behavior has been established, it is very difficult for the person to change it.

- AS causes many to understand the world from just their personal perspective. People with AS tend to have problems with understanding that others have thoughts and feelings of their own; this gets in the way of someone with AS being able to see another's perspective.

- AS often causes the person to interpret an NT's attempt to explain his or her side of the story as a criticism and "dismiss" it. As a result, the person with AS will have no way to learn from problems that occur with others and change the behavior.

- AS often causes people with AS, especially men with AS, to come to a conclusion about their self-image when they are very young, which means they decide what they are like as a person. This self-image tends to be rigid; it doesn't reflect any feedback or new information, because any information that doesn't fit with this self-image is ignored or is evaluated as a putdown and dismissed.

Being aware of AS and its impact and committing to making changes where necessary are key if a person with AS is going to make adaptive changes in his or her life. Once the diagnosis has been made, the person with AS will need some help to identify behaviors that interfere with good relationships and to gain better communication skills. For many people with AS, the most effective way to do this is to find an NT with whom they have or can build a trusting relationship. By working together, it is possible for people with AS to gain an understanding of the way NTs think and feel and to increase their awareness of and to improve interpretation of nonverbal communication. Such a person may be a family member, a friend, or a professional, any of whom must be knowledgeable about AS and its implications.

Living with AS Day to Day
Living with AS often means that people with AS find the world and the people around them confusing and bewildering. One young girl with AS, when asked what she wanted to be when she grew up, replied, "a speed bump." She explained this as wanting the world to slow down—that she hated it that "things happen too fast." Other comments I've heard from individuals with AS include questions such as, "Why don't NTs say what they mean?" or "Why don't NTs talk about facts instead of people?" All of these problems with

understanding NTs create stress and other negative feelings in people with AS. Temple Grandin states in her book, *Animals in Translation,* that fear is her main emotion. Many with AS describe their usual emotional state, especially when around others or in new situations, as consisting of fear, anxiety, and/or confusion. There is research that shows that autism spectrum disorders do seem to cause many people to live in a state of hyper-arousal—a sort of prepanic state that can be very debilitating. And, in fact, many people with AS complain of tiredness and physical ailments such as chronic muscle pain. These symptoms are often associated with stress and may get in the way of individuals with AS doing the things that they want to do because they are always feeling fatigued.

The Stress of Coping with New Situations

"I just don't get it. We've had this trip to North Carolina to buy new furniture planned for months now. In fact, it was your idea. You told me we should get the furniture here because we could get such a great discount." Sandra was unhappy because Kevin didn't want to get out of the car to go into the furniture store with her.

Kevin replied, "I don't know what's wrong. I had a good night's sleep, but I'm so tired I feel sick."

Sandra left him in the car and did the shopping alone. When she came back to the car, Kevin was sound asleep in the passenger seat.

Coping with new, stressful situations on top of the chronic stress they experience often results in some people with AS not having as much stamina as their NT partners. For Kevin, the 250-mile trip over unfamiliar roads and sleeping in a hotel left him very tired; the idea of shopping and helping Sandra make decisions about furniture was more effort than he could bear.

How Can the Person with AS Cope with Anxiety?

If you have AS, it is important to understand and recognize that there is a need to pace yourself if you experience a lot of anxiety. It's helpful, for example, to understand that certain circumstances, such as having to be around large numbers of people or finding your way in a strange town, may be extremely demanding for you because there is so much stimulation to process. Also, there is so much about the situation that is unknown, it's impossible to anticipate what you'll have to handle next. It's important to tell your partner or companions if you start feeling tired or overwhelmed. Being exhausted greatly increases the chance of miscommunication and misunderstanding, and for someone with AS, there is the risk of an extreme emotional reaction that may include lashing out at others. If both of you understand that coping with AS can be very tiring and that dealing with new situations will probably intensify your anxiety, you and your partner can take this into account when making plans.

Chronic Stress Means Less Emotional Resilience

This chronic high level of arousal also means that people with AS have a lower tolerance for and less resilience in dealing with both their own and others' emotions. This is especially true for negative feelings, such as anger and frustration. This lack of resilience often results in emotional outbursts by people with AS that, from the view of the observer, are way out of proportion to the situation. If the NT does not understand that the person with AS may be chronically over-aroused physiologically, have a lower tolerance for stress, and lack the skill to deal easily with his or her feelings, the NT may be shocked at the degree of reaction from the person with AS and judge the person unfairly.

AS-NT Differences in Recovery from Emotional Outbursts

As you think about AS-NT relationships, it's important to keep in mind that even if the NT understands that the person with AS may be prone to these emotional outbursts, these episodes are still likely to be very upsetting to the NT. It will probably take the NT a while to get over them. This is especially the case if the person with AS has lashed out at or attacked the NT. For the person with AS, once the outburst has run its course, he will have said or done what he needed to do to get the issue out of his system and will move on and behave as though nothing has happened. It is likely to take the NT much longer to get over the attack. But, as we have noted many times in this book, people with AS usually are not aware of the impact of their behavior on others, and as a result, they will not understand why the NT is still upset.

The differences in the understanding of the situation and the recovery time between the AS and the NT often results in the person with AS becoming annoyed if the NT continues to be upset or wants to discuss what happened. The NT finds this frustrating and hard to cope with and is usually left with feelings of anger. The situation becomes yet one more occasion of pain and misunderstanding to plague the relationship.

An AS Response to Being Overtired and Overstressed

Lillian and Manny were standing on the back deck of the cruise ship on which they were vacationing, waiting for the astronomy lecture that was scheduled. They were both interested in the subject and had decided to stay up for the lecture. It had been a long day though; first the flight to Miami, the taxi to the dock, and then dinner with four passengers they did not know at the required table for six. "Are you sure that the lecturer is an astronomer?" Lillian asked Manny.

"That's what the folder said, but if he isn't, I'll give the talk. Probably nobody on this ship knows anything about astronomy anyway," Manny said jokingly.

"How can you say something so stupid?" Lillian lashed out. She began to shout at Manny, "You are ignorant. You don't know anything about these people. You never met any of them until tonight, so you don't know what they know!" Manny was embarrassed and tried to quiet his wife. But Lillian, who has AS, continued to shout at him. Finally, she turned and went back to their cabin. When Manny came in a while later, she calmly inquired, "Did you enjoy the lecture?" Manny, still upset, stepped out on their balcony, shaking his head.

Lillian was clearly overstressed by the situation. There was too much information, there were too many new people, and the day had been physically tiring. It became too much for her to manage. It's not unusual for an overtired or overstressed person with AS to get angry and yell and scream over some minor incident. When Manny tried to joke with her, Lillian became angry, lost control, and lashed out at Manny. Lillian's outburst ran its course, and as far as she was concerned, the episode was over when she returned to their room. She promptly forgot about it. Lillian was not aware of the impact of her behavior on Manny and behaved toward him as if nothing had happened when he returned to their room. Manny was still shaken; he didn't understand why Lillian had verbally attacked him or why she was acting as if nothing had happened.

What Are Ways to Cope with Exhaustion and Stress?

1. If you have AS, watch out for being too stimulated or overtired! These are times you are more likely to over-respond and lose control.
2. Take a time out—get away by yourself and get some recovery time.
3. If you are NT, recognize the signs of an overloaded nervous system in people with AS, and give them space and privacy.

Stress and 'Special Interests'

Amanda, her husband Matt, and their guests Kay and Larry were sitting on the porch after dinner having coffee. Amanda and Kay had been college roommates, but they hadn't seen each other since Amanda's marriage. Kay and Larry had stopped to visit and spend the night with Amanda and Matt on their way to see Larry's family in Richmond. Matt had seemed restless, and when the conversation turned to a discussion of marital problems that a mutual friend was having, Matt stood up and left, without saying a word. In minutes, Matt returned, and without even an "excuse me," he opened a book he had been reading on genetics and began to read out loud. Kay and her husband were very surprised and looked at Amanda to try to understand what was happening. Amanda was terribly embarrassed by what she saw as Matt's rude behavior. Amanda didn't understand yet about Matt's AS and was very upset and confused by what was happening. Amanda didn't know that when someone with AS becomes overwhelmed, it is a common response to turn to their special interest. (In Chapter Two, you may remember Annie wanting to turn a stressful conversation to a monologue about her computer game characters.)

Changes in routine and having to spend extended time with others, especially people they do not know, are often struggles for individuals with AS. In such times of stress, for many individuals with AS, the need to engage in their "special interest" increases significantly. Being involved with the special interest helps the person with AS to feel more comfortable and in control. In this situation, Matt's stress level was very high; not only did they have guests, but because the guests were staying overnight, his routines would be disrupted.

Matt is not comfortable discussing emotional issues, and when the conversation turned to a discussion of the friend's marriage problems, he could no longer deal with the situation. He got up from the group and went to get the book he was reading on genetics, an area in which he was passionately interested. By bringing the book back and reading to the group, he was able to shut down the conversation about emotional topics. He felt more comfortable and in control. Amanda, not understanding that this was Matt's attempt to manage his anxiety, was embarrassed, and their guests, who had no idea what was going on, were uncomfortable.

How Can the Person with AS Cope with Stressful Situations?
Once again, being aware that changes in routine (houseguests in this case) can trigger stress means that a person with AS can plan to excuse himself early and seek out some solitude. It's helpful to keep a journal of the things that are over stressful so the person with AS will know what to watch out for.

Understanding, Identifying, and Expressing Feelings
People with AS often have difficulty recognizing their feelings; many people with AS also report having trouble telling their feelings apart—not understanding if they are anxious, afraid, or disappointed. They can only tell that the feeling is comfortable or uncomfortable. If the feeling is uncomfortable, the person with AS may lash out angrily, often not knowing what is wrong but feeling a lot of discomfort and needing to make those around him aware of it. Not only is the lashing out a problem, but not understanding what you are feeling makes it harder to identify what is causing the feeling. Being able to understand what you are feeling is critical to learning how to manage your feelings and gain emotional competence. Because many people with AS are

not able to recognize what they are feeling, it is harder for them to learn to manage their emotions. It's encouraging to know that a number of people with AS report that, over the years, they have gotten better at recognizing what they are feeling and why they are feeling it; as a result, they feel more competent to deal with their feelings.

The Other Side of the Emotional Coin: A Lack of Feelings

In contrast to people with AS who might not understand what they are feeling but are very aware they are feeling something and do express it, there are people with AS who seldom reveal their feelings or are not aware of experiencing any feelings. One man with AS reported that he felt like he just watched life but took no part in it. Asked about his emotions, he simply responded, "I don't think I have any." A successful businessman who had been diagnosed with AS a few months earlier wondered during a session if that was why he never felt anything. He had described many times that doing business deals was easy for him because he never got emotional, unlike some of the other business people with whom he dealt. I knew his mother had died recently, and I asked him about his reaction to her death. His response was to tell me that he was used to calling her once a week. He said he still thought about reaching for the phone to call her on Sunday evening, but that it was like trying to change a habit, like quitting smoking. When I pressed further, he commented that he just didn't feel anything, but that he did find himself thinking about not having to send her a check every month anymore. I knew that he had been very generous to his mother and treated her considerately, but as he described it, it seemed that although he felt very responsible for her, he didn't feel close to her or to anyone else he ever mentioned.

AS and Problems Expressing Emotions

Another issue about feelings some people with AS say they have is not only not being clear about what they are feeling, but more importantly, not knowing how to express feelings. Another man with AS told me that he didn't express his feelings because he feared that, if he did, he would lose control. But, he complained, even if he didn't say anything about what he was feeling, he and his wife would have problems anyway. He gave the following example. Twice, he had been transferred because of his work, and he and his wife had to buy a house at the new location. Even though each time he thought the house was okay and the prices of the houses were within their price range, he found himself feeling very uneasy. He didn't understand what was wrong, but he felt very uncomfortable. Instead of sharing his wife's pleasure that they had found a nice house, on each of those occasions, he retreated to bed as soon as they returned to their hotel room and wouldn't talk. Each time his wife had become quite upset and concerned about him. When she asked him what was wrong, he refused to answer. Because he didn't understand what he was feeling and didn't know how to tell her that, he just wouldn't say anything. He just knew he didn't feel right. His wife became upset.

His wife had no idea what was going on—all she knew was that he wouldn't talk to her. She worried that he was angry, but she had no idea why. She tried a number of times to get him to talk, but he refused to say anything. She grew more and more upset, and since she couldn't explain his behavior any other way, she finally assumed that he must be angry because he did not want the house they had bought. Not able to get any information from him, she cancelled the contract. He had no idea why his wife was so upset, or why she had cancelled the contract, but he was annoyed that she had done so. It meant that they needed to continue to look for a place to live. From his perspective, he had stayed in control—that was what mattered to him—and he was not aware of the impact of his behavior on his wife. He didn't understand that because he had refused to talk as a way keeping himself in control, he had left his wife so bewildered and worried that she had ended up canceling the contract on the house.

What Are Ways to Improve Emotional Competence?

Emotional competence, the ability to understand and express feelings, is a skill, and with time and the help of someone trustworthy, people with AS can gain skill at identifying and expressing some of what they are feeling. An NT can help by calling the attention of people with AS to behaviors that are likely to be indicators that they are reacting to something. For example, if the person with AS is pacing or clenching his fists, the NT should mention it and ask the person with AS to think about what he is feeling and what may be causing the feeling. The person with AS can also use the ways in which the NT responds to emotions as a model for his own behavior.

AS and Compassion

Many people with AS are quite compassionate. Dictionaries define compassion as "the ability to sympathize, or to have feelings in common." Many individuals with AS have sympathy for people that they see as underdogs or the victims of injustice. This is probably because many people with AS have themselves had experience with being mistreated by others. Growing up, they

THE AS CONCERN FOR INJUSTICE

Ever since he got his first job, Alex has been giving money to a charity that supports orphaned children around the world. He describes how helping someone "who didn't get a chance" makes him feel good.

Sharon, a New York City lawyer, spent so much of her time fighting for the homeless people in the city that she almost went bankrupt.

Eugene volunteered to be a subject in a trial for an AIDS vaccine that was being tested because of his strong feeling that gay men and women are mistreated.

Alex, Sharon, and Eugene all have AS. When asked why they did what they did, each responded that the world is very unfair and that they felt they had to do something to help people who have been mistreated.

may have been bullied because of their problems with social interaction. Because people with AS may have trouble understanding others and others' motivations, they can be naive and may be taken advantage of. Their obsession with their special interest and the lack of ability to recognize when others do not want to hear about it can result in teasing or rejection. If we add to that the fact that people with AS tend to have very long memories for experiences when they have felt mistreated and usually find it hard to forgive or forget, it is easy to see why they would sympathize greatly with those whom they believe are not treated fairly.

Using Feelings of Compassion to Improve Interpersonal Understanding

Compassion differs from empathy. Empathy is the ability to recognize and understand others' state of mind and feelings when they are different from your own. This is a skill area that is compromised in AS and is an area of functioning that can be difficult to help someone with AS understand. In her book, *Aspergers in Love,* Maxine Aston, a U.K. expert in counseling AS-NT couples, describes using the capacity for compassion to help people with AS relate better to their partners. By linking the impact of an AS behavior on a partner to the impact of an experience the person with AS has gone through, Aston helps develop an understanding of the impact of this behavior in the mind of the person with AS. For example, if the person with AS has been upset because a boss consistently overrules his decisions about projects, it is useful for a therapist to point out to the person with AS that the way he feels when that happens is the way his spouse feels when she is consistently overruled on decisions about finances.

AS and Bargaining Behavior

The AS individual's concerns about justice and fairness sometimes lead to a particular behavior pattern that can be very frustrating to an NT partner. We often hear from an NT spouse that the AS partner doesn't want to do anything without bargaining for something in return. Many people with AS are not motivated to please others and, as a result, are not willing to do things unless they are getting something in return. For example, if the NT partner asks the person with AS to empty the dishwasher, the person with AS might insist that he will only do it if the NT does something in return, such as pick up his dry cleaning. The NT partner can become very upset at this tit-for-tat behavior, where any request for help is met with a demand for something in return.

Managing Bargaining in an AS-NT Relationship

NTs who live with AS in their midst should set limits and insist that the person with AS look at a bigger picture. Relationships involve how people treat each other over time; they are not based on cutting moment-to-moment "deals." One problem that can contribute to the bargaining mentality is that many people with AS, while they may have an unusual memory for facts or things that interest them, have poor short-term memory for certain things. Unless he is interested in doing so, the person with AS

A WORD OF CAUTION ABOUT COUPLES THERAPY

Author Maxine Aston makes the point that any thera-peutic work with couples that involves AS is usually successful only if the person with AS has accepted the diagnosis and is committed to making the relationship work. Otherwise, because of the nature of AS (lack of understanding the impact of behavior on others, the "mind blindness" mentioned earlier), the person with AS will hear any attempt to get him to see his behavior to the NT as hurtful as unjust criticism and will often re-fuse to listen. If, however, the individual understands the diagnosis, it can be accepted as an opportunity to learn different behaviors to improve the relationship.

will not even register in short-term memory the fact that the NT does many activities such as cooking meals, getting laundry done, and paying bills. All these contributions made by the NT will likely not be noticed and will never be filed in the AS person's long-term memory. As a result, the person with AS feels any request to do something should be reciprocated by the NT doing something for him in return. It can be useful for the NT to write down a list of his or her contributions to making things work.

Don't say it—it probably won't be heard. It is usually easier for people with AS to process something if they read it, rather than listening to a long list of items.

Understanding Other AS Traits: Tenacity and Control
Tenacity in AS Individuals

Tenacity in AS is the good news and the bad news. It's not clear just what causes tenacity in individuals with AS, but as one parent of an adult with AS said, "Boy, I know it when I see it!" It is not unusual that when individuals with AS make up their minds about something, it is difficult, if not impossible, for others to change their minds, or even for them to change their own minds. One man with AS who had decided he was going to divorce his wife stated, "I know I may be doing the wrong thing. But I know that once I've decided to do something, it's impossible for me not to do it." It was obvious from the man's statement that he felt incapable of changing his mind once he got started on a certain path. This difficulty with changing a thought pattern (sometimes referred to as perseveration) may be a part of the biological differences in the AS brain. Perseveration is common in certain other medical conditions that involve the brain.

This tenacity can be very adaptive if it is directed toward solving difficult problems, especially in the world of research or work. A successful researcher who worked in computer science once told us that when he had a particularly difficult or complex program to develop, he was unable to think of anything else and that people around him often had to remind him to stop to eat. Even leaving his office to sleep became intolerable, and he finally resorted to bringing in a sleeping bag to his office. This compulsive behavior, unlike that seen in people with obsessive-compulsive disorder, is not reported by the person with AS as causing distress. It seems instead to be a highly energized, motivated experience.

Control Issues
"Everything has to be his way!" When we've worked together in therapy for a good while and when a sense of trust has developed, AS-NT couples I've worked with can sometimes develop a sense of humor about this refrain. One man with AS, who had a dry sense of humor, used to mutter it under his breath when his wife was talking. When questioned, he responded, "I'm meditating. It's my mantra. Everything has to be his way!" As people with AS and those around them gain an understanding of the syndrome, the "mantra" begins to make sense. People with AS, probably as a result of certain cognitive processing problems, have trouble with change and long for predictability. By being in "control," or having things their way, their anxiety level drops, and they can feel some level of comfort and relief.

What Are Ways to Cope with AS Individuals
Wanting to Control Things?
People with AS and those around them benefit greatly by understanding what is behind this need for control. They can then develop better ways to manage it. Here are some ideas from AS-NT couples with whom I've worked:

Try to identify what purpose the control is serving.

THE QUESTION:

1. Is the purpose to avoid something like having to deal with un-familiar guests?

2. Is the purpose to keep something comforting in place (like re-fusing to give up a tatty, old, but familiar recliner)?

3. Is the purpose to keep control of everyone around you?

THE RESPONSE:

1. Life with AS or an individual with AS requires a lot of com-promise. This is a good place to practice compromising! What priority does this social situation have on a scale of 1 (low) to 5 (high) for either party? Don't say the priority number; write it down (like a secret ballot), and set a limit on the number of 5 (most important) items in any month that either partner can claim.

2. If that chair has got to go, let the person with AS select the new one to make sure that it is comfortable.

3. There are times for giving in, times for compromise, and times for setting limits. No one person who lives with others can always have it his way. Having AS is not a ticket to always getting your way. When people live together or are in rela-tionships, everyone's needs count. So it is critical to not let the

AS-driven need dominate the household. It can be difficult for people with AS to change a behavior pattern once set. So it's best to set this limit on controlling behavior at the beginning of the relationship.

"I don't want to go to Barbados for a vacation. I don't like foreign countries, even if they are islands. I think we should get a place at Myrtle Beach."

"I'm tired of doing the same thing every year. If we go to Barbados, we'll be able to try some new things like snorkeling or scuba diving."

Many NTs like change and even adventure; they use their time off as an opportunity to try something new—to break up the routine or even the monotony of everyday life. It is different for people with AS. Most like the known and prefer routine, because to them, routine represents safety and comfort. It's important that the NT's wishes and needs get addressed fairly if the relationship is to be a success. If the person with NT gives in constantly to the person with AS, he or she will almost certainly develop feelings of resentment. At the same time, the person with AS will become more and more controlling.

Risk Aversion and AS

Why are so many people with AS so averse to trying something new? Trying something new usually represents a risk to someone with AS. And risk to AS individuals goes against the fabric of their being. Why?

- **Many people with AS feel a need to be perfect and for others to see them as perfect.** This is probably a way to guard against the feelings of low self-esteem to which many people with AS are vulnerable. Trying something new means they probably won't be able to perform perfectly and, as a result, they will be uncomfortable.

- **Many people with AS do struggle with low self-esteem,** and low self-esteem undermines the self-confidence required to try something new.

- **Fear of failure often drives people with AS unmercifully.** A successful executive with AS, when asked what motivated him to achieve so much in his career, responded, "I've never been motivated to achieve anything. I've never understood people who set goals and then went about them. My whole life has been based on the fear of failure. That's why I am where I am." For someone with AS, agreeing to try something new can feel like setting themselves up for failure.

There are of course other reasons for people with AS to be unwilling to try something new. If the person has a narrow fixed interest such as is common in AS, he or she may have absolutely no interest or willingness to do anything else. One woman with AS had an all-consuming interest in collecting lichen that grew only above a certain elevation in the Rocky Mountains. She and her husband had spent every vacation there for the thirty-one years they have been married. She had no interest in any of the things her husband suggested that they might do for a change and insisted instead that they do what interested her.

In a number of cases of AS, there is a lack of curiosity and the drive to explore that for NTs is usually present from childhood. This may be related to the neurological differences present in AS. In other cases, where there is resistance to trying something new, it may reflect the need to control change to avoid being stressed. However, as some people with AS gain life experience, they may be more willing to try new things. If their experience is a good one, they may be encouraged to experiment further. Some people with AS have told us that learning to tolerate some risk has made their lives much more interesting.

How Can a Person with AS Learn to Deal with Risk?
If you have AS, it can make your life richer if you learn how to manage some risk. Here are some steps to begin to feel more comfortable with idea of trying something new:

1. Ask yourself what's the worst that can happen?
2. If the worst does happen, what could I do? Who could help?
3. Remind yourself that everyone has a learning curve in new situations and that it is natural to need time to be comfortable with something new.

Branching out and trying something new can make your life interesting and more satisfying. As teenagers might say, "Try it, (maybe) you'll like it!"

Impulsive Behavior and AS

Occasionally, we will meet people with AS who, instead of managing their life by doing things to control their experience, will respond to their internal anxiety and external stress by behaving impulsively. In her book, *Loving Mr. Spock,* Barbara Jacobs draws a very powerful portrait of Danny, the AS man she loved and with whom she lived for a long time. His solution to situations that began to tumble into disasters was to drop whatever he was doing and throw himself into some new venture or to seek a geographical solution by moving to a new location to escape the problem. In Chapter Three, we discussed problems with executive function that are often a part of the AS symptom profile and that can negatively affect the ability to make a plan and execute it effectively. This difficulty in thinking through and completing a plan of action can mean that people with AS, while they may have very good ideas for their work or their personal life, will not be able to execute these ideas. The plan is not thought through, and the individual cannot figure out or follow through on what it would take for the plan to be successful. The efforts fall apart, sometimes creating quite problematic situations. In an attempt to regain some sort of control, the person with AS may impulsively jump into something else or move off to some other place to try for a new start.

Unfortunately, the same AS-associated difficulties that started the cycle usually make the new situation even more difficult. All of the change and all the new learning and understanding required to cope with new situations make the challenge to the person with AS more severe or even impossible. It is almost certain that the person will fail, and the cycle of impulsively running off or starting something new will repeat itself again.

John was very angry and frightened. I had been assigned as his therapist for the period of time he was in the hospital, and we were meeting for the first time. I knew he had been given a choice of going into a psychiatric hospital or having charges brought against him for harassing a woman with whom he worked. "John, can you tell me about yourself and how you came to be here?" I asked.

"It's not fair that I was forced to come here. My boss never gave me a chance to prove myself," replied John.

"What did you want to prove?"

The question opened the door to a long and poignant story of a man who was unquestionably brilliant. John worked in the computer systems part of a large financial services company. He had an idea for payment transfers that his boss had acknowledged could revolutionize a part of that industry. He had been fired from a previous job in the same business, but his new boss had accepted John's explanation that it was the result of a personality conflict with his former employers. John was assigned a team to help him design and develop his new system. As the days and then weeks went by and there was no progress on the project, the workplace became very tense. John began coming in late and leaving early; it was obvious he was drinking heavily. On the day he ended up being hospitalized, he had come into work quite drunk. He began to verbally abuse and threaten the woman who provided support services for the group when she couldn't find a document he had misplaced. His boss called the police, but the assistant didn't want to press charges. She admired John and felt he had some emotional problems. She suggested that it would be better for him to get treatment than to go to jail. John's boss agreed, and John ended up in the hospital.

Over the next month, I learned that a similar scene had been played out at least three times in John's life. He would have a wonderful idea and he would find someone to support it, but John was never able to organize it and make it happen. He would then get into some kind of trouble, disappear, and move to a new town to begin the cycle once again.

It took John a long time to begin to trust me or to be able to even consider his role in what was happening. But as I pointed out, he was in the unfortunate position of choosing to trust me or the police. Not surprisingly, he said he didn't think it was much of a choice. Together we stumbled on a way to work together. I have a passion for dumb puns and so did he; we could occasionally share a laugh. It was a way to begin the work of understanding each other, an important part of doing therapy with someone who has AS. I had to translate the NT world for him and come to understand just how his AS affected him so that I could then help him to see how he was affected and how this AS-related behavior led to his difficulties. We worked together for almost five years. Much of our focus was on the value of structure and support for all of us, but especially for someone with AS, and we were able to find ways for John to get some structure into his life. Instead of living alone, he moved in with his sister, who traveled a great deal on business but basically kept the household organized. She was younger than John and had always looked up to him while at the same time being protective of him. John felt comfortable with her. This ensured that John had a stable but undemanding home life. At work, he was assigned to work with a much older colleague. This man's skills were complimentary to John's, and this colleague was able to plan and organize the effort needed to achieve John's ideas. He also acted as a mentor and made sure that John didn't have to interact much with others and didn't have to deal with people issues. John was able to concentrate on the part of the work that interested him and at which he excelled. With this structure in place, his work group was able to turn his ideas into very successful products. John joined a hiking group to keep himself busy (and away from bars) on weekends. He met Rita, who was a member of the same hiking club, and he began spending a lot of his free time with her. Rita was almost fifteen years older than him and quite self-sufficient, but she enjoyed taking care of others and was very kind to John. John, with some assistance, had put together a world filled with structure and support. We mutually decided that it was time to end the therapy. John felt that his life was in good order and stated that he no longer felt the need to run away. It seemed to me that John had enough support around him to help him deal with his life.

Summing It All Up

Harry Stack Sullivan, a psychiatrist renowned for his work with people with schizophrenia, was once asked the secret of his success.

His response was, "I never forget for a moment that we are all more human than otherwise." There is a lot of wisdom in those few words. We share our humanness and the wonder and pain that it implies, and that should be the basis for living in mutual respect. While living in an AS-NT world, respect for each other and the willingness to try to understand each other's cultures is the key to bridging our differences. Wendy Lawson, whom we mentioned in Chapter One, coined a term we find both appealing and useful. After spending some time understanding the challenges posed by having AS and recognizing that in a number of ways she related to the world around her differently than the NTs she knew, she came to see that having AS for her meant not disabilities but different abilities. She coined the word diffabilities. In a number of ways, those diffabilities make AS-NT relationships interesting but also quite difficult, and in the next two chapters, we'll look at how those difficulties play out. Not all the stories are pretty, but they will help to define the opportunities for change that can build the bridge between the two cultures.

CHAPTER EIGHT

Building Relationships and Support Systems

Dana looked at the caller ID number, which she recognized as her brother's. "Oh dear. What now?" she thought. "Hi Les. How are you?" she asked her younger brother, dreading the answer.

"I just called to tell you I got a job. I'm going to drive a taxi for Mr. Geddis. He is paying me six dollars an hour, and I'll get tips. I'll work Wednesday, Thursday, Friday, Saturday, and Sunday. I'll be working from noon to seven at night." Les went on to describe the kind of car used as a taxi in the small Pennsylvania town where he lived. When he finally stopped for breath, Dana said, "Les, that's absolutely wonderful. I'm really happy for you!"

Dana didn't want Les to get started on cars, his special interest that he studies obsessively; Les knew the make and model of every car ever built in the United States, the colors they came in, the horsepower, etc., and he loved telling everyone everything he knew. Les had become much more aware that he should not go into what the family called his "car spiel," but when he was stressed or excited, he sometimes had trouble not doing so.

"What did Dad say about your new job?" Dana asked.

"He told me that people would be relying on me, and that I had to be responsible and show up on time for work."

Dana, her father, and her two sisters knew that Les, who has AS, wanted very much to have a job and be more independent. He was thirty-five but had never held a steady job. It was difficult for him to have anyone tell him what to do, and over the years, his bosses had become tired of his arguing with them and had let him go, much to the family's concern. Les, because of his AS, had trouble understanding how his argumentative behavior resulted in his losing his job. Mr. Geddis, Les's new boss, had known the family all of Les's life. He belonged to the same church as the family and had seen Les grow up. Dana thought that it was very kind of him to give Les a chance. Dana found herself thinking that growing up in a small town had its advantages—people reached out to support one another. Mr. Geddis had given Les another chance. Hopefully, with Les's love of cars, this job might work out.

Dana wanted very much for her brother's new job to work out. She knew that he would feel better about himself if he was working, but Les often had difficulty with relationships, which made it hard for him to keep a job. He often got into disagreements with coworkers and even his boss. Mr. Geddis understood about Les's Asperger Syndrome (AS) and had tried to be supportive of him for a number of years, encouraging him to volunteer at the church. He had also found Les some hourly work several times, parking cars at the country club for weddings and christenings. Les thought of Mr. Geddis as his friend, and it was very important to Les to have a friend.

One of the ways clinicians have noted that AS differs from autism is in the desire for human contact. People with autism often show more interest in objects than in people, while many people with AS want to be with people and to have relationships. The nature of AS makes relationships difficult, however, since the core problems in AS are understanding others and difficulty with communication, especially nonverbal communication. We all differ in the extent to which relationships are important to us and the amount of effort we are willing to invest to make them work. But for people with AS, it requires more effort to be in relationships because of differences in the way their brains function.

Other AS-related issues may complicate the effort to be in a relationship. Sensory integration problems that are common in AS can make touching and physical closeness uncomfortable or even painful. The predisposition of many people with AS to be hypersensitive to criticism and to have difficulty ever accepting that they are wrong coupled with issues with self-esteem make some people with AS "prickly partners." Others may find it difficult to relate to such partners.

Learning from Relationships

Louise overheard her daughter Sophia by the front door, saying good night to Beth and Bill, old family friends who had come to the house for dinner. She was a bit surprised that Sophia was saying good night, since Sophia had not wanted to join them for dinner. In fact, Sophia had insisted on an early dinner and had spent the entire evening, while Bill and Beth were visiting, in her room studying.

"I'm so glad you came for dinner. It's nice to see you both. Let's plan to get together soon," said Sophia. It sounded odd to Louise to hear Sophia mimicking the words that she usually said when saying good night to guests, but she knew from working with her counselor that mimicry is one of the ways people with AS use to learn to navigate social situations. She was pleased, because she was aware that Sophia wanted very much to fit in and worked hard to learn how to handle social occasions.

"Thanks. We really enjoyed it. Dinner was delicious; I'll have to get your lamb recipe, Louise. Good night, Sophia," said Beth.

Louise handed her guests their coats while Sophia held the door open. Beth and Bill had known Sophia from the time she was born and understood Sophia's AS and that she occasionally would play her mother's role in social situations as she practiced her social skills.

"Good night, Louise. I'll talk to you tomorrow." Bill and Beth took their coats and walked to their car in the driveway.

It still seemed a bit strange to Louise to hear Sophia repeating phrases that she herself used, sometimes inappropriately.

Sophia had talked to Bill and Beth as though she had been the one entertaining them all evening, when Sophia had actually been in her room since before the guests had arrived. When Sophia had first started doing this, Louise had become upset, thinking her teenaged daughter was mocking her, and she often got into arguments with her daughter over this behavior. But when the fights led to Louise and Sophia seeing a therapist, they had learned from the therapist that this "social echolalia" was very common in people with AS and was in fact often very adaptive. By mimicking her mother, Sophia was practicing social skills that helped her to deal with people interactions that would otherwise be very difficult to handle. Sophia felt comfortable with Beth and Bill, who were almost like an aunt and uncle to her. Sophia had wanted to say good night to them and had relied on her memory of the way Louise handled guests' departures to say her own good nights.

Echolalia is the repeating of words or phrases (or even longer passages of speech in the case of some people with autistic spectrum disorders) of one person by another. It is usually viewed as noncommunicative or dysfunctional in the field of psychiatry, but in autistic spectrum disorders, echolalia may have a useful function. It may be used to manage stress, to indicate that the person doesn't understand, and perhaps, most importantly, to rehearse. The individual with AS may learn to copy the speech of others, even at a very complex level. The echoing often includes the cadence and intonation of the original speech and may be more expressive sounding than the usual speech of the person with AS. Unfortunately, if the diagnosis of AS in not known or understood, the echolia may be seen as mockery and be very offensive to the person being echoed. Also, in some cases, the echoing may be misleading, causing others to believe that the person with AS has better communicative skills than he or she actually has, leading to unrealistic expectations of the social abilities of this person.

Social Echolalia

Social echolalia is a phrase used to describe the imitation of another person's behavior in social situations, often without real understanding of the situation or what the behavior actually means, especially the subtleties. Sophia had not invited Beth and Bill, nor had she cooked the dinner that was served. Her mother had done all those things, and in that context, if Louise had said the words that Sophia used, they would have made sense. When Sophia, who wasn't even at dinner, had mimicked the behavior she had observed in her mother on other such occasions, it seemed strange. But the behavior was one of Sophia's coping strategies as she struggled to learn how to handle social interactions. This ability to reproduce behaviors is quite common in AS individuals from a very young age. One example is a four-year-old boy who was given a Barney costume for Halloween. He put the costume on and began singing and dancing a whole set of songs that he had seen Barney perform on television. What was interesting about this behavior was that until he put on the costume, no one had ever seen him imitating Barney or singing his songs, and his family had no idea that he had memorized them all.

Identification as a Way to Adapt

As people with AS gain life experience, many identify a series of people whom they see as powerful, successful, or accomplished (especially at something the person with AS values or wants) and adopt that person's way of dealing with the world. One young woman with AS, whom I first met as a child, had tracked very closely with a series of women, beginning when she was very young. She first began mimicking conversations that she overheard between her mother and a friend. The child would repeat in an echolalic way just who in the neighborhood was pregnant, who had miscarried "at four months," and who was having difficulty becoming pregnant. This conversation, repeated in a very grave tone of voice identical to the neighbor's, was of course completely inappropriate for a five-year-old. But as this young woman developed, her choice of role models—excellent students whose behavior she imitated—helped her to do well in school. Occasionally, the "model" friend would have a gift or talent that she did not, such as being musical or good at dance, and although she would try to follow suit, her ability to mimic would not be enough for her to be successful. She would then seek another model friend. She was, with considerable effort and by using models, able to live away at college and graduate on schedule. During her years of growing up, she would occasionally be without a model and would become more withdrawn, complain constantly of having too much schoolwork, and in general function less well. As soon as she was able to identify a new model, there would be shifts in what was important to her, based on what mattered to the newest model. This could be seen in her choice of clothing and her demands for her parents to give her whatever was the latest "in" thing, such as a pager or cell phone. Watching the modeling process in this young woman was like seeing someone act out a series of roles. The use of models on which to pattern behavior was in this case very helpful.

Females with AS are more likely to follow this pattern of social echolalia than males. It may be because of this patterning behavior that fewer females than males are diagnosed with AS. Women, as mentioned earlier, are often under more pressure to fit in than men are, and some women with AS have worked out ways to benefit from this.

The "Social Sister" Phenomenon

Perhaps a special example of this social echolalia in women is what we've come to think of as the "social sister" phenomenon. In this case, the sister with AS will imitate her NT sister's life and will follow it step by step, even including marrying and having children. The reliance of the sister with AS on her NT sister can be pretty demanding and may include the AS sister insisting on multiple contacts every day and that any free time be spent together. In cases of the social sister phenomenon, the mother is usually shut out and frequently devalued by the daughter with AS. And, in fact, it's pretty common for individuals with AS, especially females, to resent direction and advice from parents, especially mothers. This seems to be because the person with AS often hears the advice as criticism or as an act of control. Also, many people with AS, especially if they are bright, feel they are smarter than most of the people around them and feel that they know better than the people around them. In the case of the "social sister," since the high-functioning person with AS has made the choice to mimic the sibling's behavior, these issues don't come up.

Most AS experts agree that the more social experience the person with AS has, the more positive the outcome. A question remains as to whether the improvement is the result of increased social interaction or the cause of increased social interaction. It probably doesn't really matter. We all learn from practice, whether it's the piano or becoming more emotionally competent. The experience of attempting an interaction and having a good response means we are more likely to try it a second time. It seems likely that by spending more time with others, the person with AS will gradually lose some of his or her anxiety about interacting with others. This cycle can self-reinforce, and as social experience grows, the ability to handle the anxiety can grow as well.

The Value of Being Around Others

There is not a lot of research on the impact of socialization across the lifespan of individuals with AS, but we know from broader research that contact with and the support of others has beneficial results. This benefit includes not only mental health but physical health as well. The research in this area is very compelling and is one of the most powerful and consistent findings in the area of human well-being.

If we look at the opposite condition—loneliness or isolation—there is further confirmation of the value of relationships.

The British psychoanalyst John Bowlby's landmark studies of what happens to hospitalized infants separated from the care of their mother make the power of attachment, or the lack of it, very clear. The infants in these studies failed to thrive and experienced severe effects on emotional and intellectual development. At the other end of life, we know from research that when one spouse dies, the chance of the other spouse dying within the year is much higher than one might expect.

Research on loneliness has found two kinds of isolation that result in a sense of being alone. The first is social isolation, which is the result of not feeling part of any social group, or not feeling valued or important to the group. Many things can lead to social isolation, ranging from personal traits, such as severe shyness, to life events, such as divorce. For people with AS, the awareness of being different, of having trouble fitting in, all too often creates a painful sense of social isolation. The individual with AS often experiences this aloneness very keenly, and this seems to be especially true before he or she is diagnosed. The diagnosis helps people with AS understand their difference and to know that they are not alone—that others have the same differences.

The second kind of isolation is emotional isolation. This form of isolation may lead to depression. Emotional isolation involves the sense of not having any close relationships with other people. In the case of AS, although many people with AS do like to be with people, the nature of these attachments is not clear, and it is not apparent how strong these attachments are. As a result, it is unknown whether these relationships are as helpful in warding off the sense of emotional isolation in people with AS as they are in NTs. Many times, people with AS seem to recover from the grief of losing a family member or spouse more quickly than NTs and often will quickly move on to another relationship that will serve their needs. It is not clear what this behavior implies, but it may reflect a more practical rather than emotional view of relationships on the part of the person with AS.

Advice for Dealing with Social and Emotional Isolation

• **Social Isolation.** For people with AS, understanding that their difficulties are the result of neurobiological differences and that others have the same differences is helpful in feeling less socially isolated. For many people with AS, the Internet has been a blessing. Through the Internet, people with AS can easily contact others with the same differences and share thoughts and experiences without the intensity of face-to-face interaction. The Internet has many Web sites set up by individuals with AS, and there are chat rooms dedicated to individuals with AS. This virtual community is a good place to learn how others get their need to belong fulfilled.

• **Emotional Isolation.** The second source of loneliness is emotional loneliness and is the result of not feeling connected to any other person, especially in an emotionally close way. We don't fully understand the role of emotion in the life of people with AS, but there's a lot of evidence to suggest that there is a need to feel important to others and to have their approval. One man with AS who had married twice, had divorced twice, and was now in a third relationship said in talking about his marital history that it was important to him for his wife to admire him and to treat him with "unconditional positive regard." For him, that was the fundamental condition to having a relationship with a woman, and he was continuing his search to find a relationship that met those conditions. Although we all want to be liked and admired, insisting on unconditional positive regard is too much to ask of a partner. Having an unrealistic, naive view of relationships almost always leads to chronic disappointment, and bitterness toward people and relationships is likely to develop. A good mental health plan is to write down your expectations about relationships and what your experiences in relationships have been with regard to those expectations, and look for patterns. If you find that your friends or partners consistently disappoint you, it's important to question whether your expectations are realistic, as well as whether or not you are registering all the things that others do for you because they care for you.

How Can We Develop Good Relationships?
For people with AS, gaining understanding of friendship is a good first step toward developing relationships. As trite as it may sound, we all benefit by keeping in mind that good relationships begin with the golden rule: Treat others as you would like them to treat you. In a way, it's a tall order because it requires that we treat others with tolerance and respect and be aware and appreciative when they reciprocate. It's important to understand that one-sided relationships won't work.

When we are looking to establish relationships, one of the first requirements is to find places we can meet people. Here are some ideas:

1. **Follow your passion.** If building model railroad layouts is what you enjoy, find a club (the Internet's a good place to look, or look in hobby magazines that focus on your passion) and tap into a group that shares your interest. The shared interest makes conversation, and eventually perhaps relating, easier.

2. **Look for organized activities, even if you are only a little bit interested.** Playing in a softball league or learning yoga are opportunities to get to know people in more structured, less intense ways.

3. **Volunteer and then volunteer again.** Maybe you have an interest in music, and your church choir needs someone to catalog music, schedule practice, and so on. Or perhaps you enjoy working with the elderly—you can volunteer at a local nursing home and be most welcome.

   Volunteering has a number of advantages, including making you feel better about yourself for doing something good for others. It gives you a chance to spend time with other volunteers, and people who volunteer tend to be kind, caring people who are quite accepting. And of course volunteering offers an opportunity to help the underdog or bring about more social justice—two themes that are important to many people with AS.

Shy Gorillas

One subset of people with AS have particular difficulty in relating to other people. This is the group, described in Chapter Two, that is often diagnosed as having schizoid personality disorder. The core symptoms seen in this condition include emotional detachment, social isolation, poor empathy, odd communication, and obsessive interests. These symptoms sound very familiar, don't they? The core symptoms are the same as those of the autistic spectrum disorders, and many clinicians who are familiar with autistic spectrum disorders believe that eventually this diagnostic category will be folded into AS. However, one thing sets this group apart from others with AS. They are quite distrustful, even paranoid, and profoundly shy, so much so that it is rare for them to socialize or to have relationships except with others like themselves. Observing this, Dr. John Ratey, who, along with Catherine Johnson, wrote the book *Shadow Syndromes,* describes himself as being reminded of the extremely shy gorillas observed and studied for so many years by Dian Fossey. In writing about this group of patients, Dr. Ratey has characterized them as "shy gorillas" as a way of acknowledging their extreme need for remoteness and privacy. Dr. Ratey's shy gorillas are a remarkable group, with IQs ranging in the 160s, and unlike as is usually the case in AS, where the majority are male, the majority of shy gorillas are female. None of Dr. Ratey's patients were married, and all were extremely successful in their careers. Dr. Ratey remarked that with this group of patients, he always felt like an observer and that direct contact did not seem possible.

There is one symptom common to the shy gorillas that is not seen as often in the rest of the AS group, and that is paranoia. A number of people with AS have some degree of mistrust of others, probably as a result of painful experiences in relationships, but in general, they are usually not paranoid in the way that shy gorillas are. Shy gorillas are actually afraid of people; as a result, it is very difficult for anyone to get close to them, and they are quick to withdraw if something disturbs them in the relationship.

Dr. Francisca Happe, a U.K. autism researcher, offers a compelling explanation for the paranoia of this special group of people who likely have AS. Dr. Happe's theory is that the remarkable intelligence of this group has in one way worked against them, because they, more than others with AS, are aware that others have minds of their own. They have used their powerful intellect to work out and come to an understanding that others have minds of their own, but there are two very serious problems with this. First, by the time the shy gorilla has developed a theory of mind, he or she probably has experienced a childhood filled with stress and anxiety trying to understand relationships. People with AS, you will remember, process information about people and emotions using a different area of the brain than NTs. That means that their processing requires a lot more effort, and it is easier to misinterpret their experience. Shy gorillas, because of their profound shyness and sensitivity, are likely to have many negative interpretations of situations that other people would see as neutral or even positive. As a result of their shyness and the fact that they lack the easy, automatic processing of social information that the NT has, there are far too many opportunities for these shy gorillas to "get it wrong." They seem biased to misinterpret their experience in a negative way and have concluded that people are bad and frightening. So while shy gorillas may have relatively well-developed theories of mind, instead of having improved social skills, they have become paranoid.

The second problem faced by this group is that while they do understand that others have thoughts and feelings of their own, and they may even at times read these thoughts and feelings right, more often than not, their reading of the thoughts and feelings of others is wrong. The problem is that because they are so intellectually gifted, and in matters of fact and logic are usually right, they are completely confident that their perceptions are right. What's more, they even consider themselves to be exceptionally capable of empathy, or, put another way, they believe that they have outstanding abilities in reading others. The result is that these brilliant people seem to have a dark view of humanity and will probably never be willing (or able) to question the conclusions they have drawn. So, while many of these extraordinary, high-functioning people may long for contact, because of their fear and negative view of people and their shyness, they will likely find attempts to have a relationship intolerable.

Support Systems: Making Them Work for You

A good support system helps us feel less lonesome and isolated and helps us to do a better job of managing the challenges life invariably throws our way. As adults, that means we have relationships with a number of people that we can look to when we need support. Here are some possibilities, in order of the different life stages: 1. Parents, 2. Siblings, 3. Friends, 4. Spouse, 5. The waitress at the diner.

There are a couple of key things for the person with AS to keep in mind if he or she is trying to establish a successful support system.

- **Rely on yourself to seek support.** If it's Saturday morning, you're lonely, and everyone you know has plans, instead of withdrawing and staying in bed or playing your 5,000th game of computer solitaire, get yourself to the diner for a cup of coffee or a hot chocolate. Practice just smiling when you order and thanking your server with another smile. "Have a nice day" goes well with paying the check. There's no need for any big conversation. If you repeat this ritual several weeks in a row, you'll most likely get a warm smile of recognition that will help you feel more grounded and ready to deal with the day.

- **Seek help on problems at work.** Are you having a problem with your boss or a coworker, or are you just trying to better organize your work? Think a bit about a person on your support system list that is most likely to have some knowledge about your line of work and who will be able to help you. Seek that person out for some ideas on how to deal with the problem.

- **Make notes before going into a discussion.** Sometimes it's hard for someone to get started talking about something that is bothering them. A small pad of paper or 3 x 5 index cards are great places to write down the key elements of the problem. Writing your thoughts down will help you make sure you don't leave something important out. (Also, jot down the ideas that were discussed. This will ensure that you don't forget anything important about what's been said.)

- **Don't abuse your support system!** As adults, we all have to learn how to use a support system. Although we must assume responsibility for ourselves, we can use our support system for guidance, feedback, and a sounding board. But everyone in the support system has his or her own life, so don't expect too much. These individuals can't solve or take care of your problems for you. Also, don't make too many demands on any one person, or he or she may find being your friend too draining.

Here is a word of caution about selecting your support system. Unfortunately, not everyone can be trusted, and it's helpful to learn a little bit about people with whom you might consider striking up a friendship. Do they seem to have pretty well-established lives? Do they have other friends? Do you know people who know them? Sometimes people with AS tend to trust easily—a very nice quality—but there will occasionally be people who will take advantage of this trustworthiness.

Putting Together a Support System

A support system gives us a set of relationships that we can depend on for different kinds of help. While the idea of a support system seems pretty simple, it's sometimes hard for us to get it all figured out. How do we know who to go to for what? What if we find ourselves so upset we can't think straight? There is a tool that can be helpful for sorting this all out.

Some years ago, I was working in a psychiatric hospital, and insurance companies were pressuring the staff to discharge patients after very short stays. This was causing concern for staff and patients alike. How could we make the transition from the hospital support system to dealing with the outside world go better? We decided to do a brainstorming session at the next patient-staff meeting.

At the beginning of the meeting, it seemed only the staff was participating, but after some laughs about some wildly implausible suggestions, everyone began to participate, and a plan began to take shape. It started with a suggestion by an art therapist that everyone draw their world outside the hospital. Amid complaints of "I can't do that; I can't draw," a young man who had been quiet during most of his time on the ward volunteered, "I have an idea." He walked up to the chalkboard and drew two circles. He labeled one work and another school. His idea was to list whom he could turn to for help when he needed it in either of those situations.

The rest of the group insisted he add a third circle for social situations (a tough place for a lot of us to deal with!). The group picked up the idea, and everyone agreed to draw their own "field analysis," the name assigned to the drawings. As the group began to get involved with the idea, they began to add more information, such as what it is ok to ask for—parents for financial support, siblings for rides when needed, friends for emotional support. The group decided they should add telephone numbers to make it easier to reach out when they needed help.

For many in the group, it was the first time they had ever really thought about how many people there were around them from whom they could expect some level of support. For others, they began to recognize "holes" in their support system, and there were conversations both with therapists and in the ward community about how to go about finding people who could fill the spaces.

The last stage of the field analysis was to identify what the patient could give in exchange. Amid occasional bouts of hilarity, in response to certain ideas such as, "My therapist will get a chance to see my handsome face once a week!" everyone in the group began, often with the help of others, to identify things about themselves that others valued. The field analysis diagram became a useful tool to help the group keep a hopeful perspective on their future. It might be worthwhile for you to consider doing your own field analysis.

Key Elements of the Support System
Parents

If you are lucky enough to still have parents around, they can be one of your best sources of support. Parents come in all shapes, sizes, and personalities, but in most cases, parents really do want to do what is best for their children, even if their children are now adults. And most parents are more than willing to help their offspring when they can, especially if they know that their child is dealing with some sort of problem. It can be very hard on parents to know that an offspring has some neurological differences that may make life more difficult, and it's very common for the parents to feel guilt that they are somehow responsible for their child's problem. When the problem the person with AS has is difficulty dealing with human relationships, especially in today's psychologically minded age, parents fear that they must have done something wrong in rearing their child.

In addition, the emotional distance that is fairly common in the person with AS often makes parents feel that they may have failed their child or that the parent is not loved or is not lovable. Often the opportunity to be helpful gives the parent a chance to feel that they are making up for anything they may have done to contribute to their child's problem and feel closer.

We know that it is not uncommon for someone with AS to have a parent with some AS characteristics themselves. Having these AS characteristics may help the parent understand the child with AS more easily and can be very valuable in helping the child learn how to cope better. Sometimes the attachment behavior of the AS child becomes so intense that the non-AS parent is excluded. It's important to find a way that both parents are involved with helping and being a part of the child's life.

Having a long family history where AS has been present for a number of generations but the AS diagnosis has never been made often means there have been many emotionally upsetting incidents and a lot of stress in the family system. As a result of this history, parents may be at times overprotective or have difficulty having realistic expectations of their child, even into adulthood. It's important to have appropriate expectations of the person with AS if this person is to reach his or her potential. When the diagnosis of AS is finally made, the family would likely benefit by having some professional help in understanding what is the right level of expectation for that particular person with AS.

Another important problem to understand is that individuals with AS tend to think of advice, or even someone trying to explain their point of view, as criticism, and they often become resentful. This situation is especially true in women with AS, who frequently express anger that their parents want to "baby them" or that their parents are overprotective.

What Are Ways that Families Can Deal with AS?

• Once the diagnosis has been made and accepted, the family can begin the process of learning about AS and the different kinds of problems and abilities associated with it. This information makes it possible to figure out how to be most helpful, so it is very important for the family to understand the nature of AS by reading about it, talking to professionals, and being in contact with other families that have AS in their midst. As a result of their diagnosis and learning about the condition, people with AS may begin to understand that they are prone to hearing instructions or criticism even when it is not there. The person with AS is then better able, through use of logical thinking, to listen for and work out what is really being said.

• Someone once said, "Raising children is the price you pay for being raised." Although this is a clever thought, it's an awfully long-term view and a rather negative one at that. An expression of appreciation in both directions seems much more appropriate and can go a long way toward making a relationship more valuable. A simple "Thanks for all you do for me, Mom and Dad" or "I am proud of you. You are a good person" can go a long way toward making the relationship better for all concerned.

Siblings

Sibling relationships, whether there is the issue of AS or not, in many cases tend to frequently swing between the extremes of love and hate while children are growing up. "Rivalry," "hero-worship," "bickering," and "protecting from others" are all words and phrases that are recalled when we think about sibling relationships. Having a child with AS can make family life more complicated for all the siblings. If one member of a family has different or special needs, it can be hard for the other children to understand. It can, and often does, feel as if the different child gets his or her way all the time or is the favored one. These wounds can last a very long time, and often the healing only begins if there is the understanding that comes with a diagnosis. There is also sometimes a history of the child with AS abusing siblings. AS can cause a great deal of frustration in the affected child, and he or she may lash out at an NT sibling who is claiming time, attention, or a toy that the AS child is not prepared to share. If AS children direct their rage toward NT children and physically attack them, it is critically important that parents stop this behavior immediately. In adulthood, if there is a history of abuse toward a sibling, parents and the person with AS need to express their regrets.

How Can Sibling Relationships Help in AS?

If the family functions well, having siblings can be of benefit to both the AS and NT siblings.

- **Individuals with AS can use a sibling near their age as a role model.** They can learn from siblings how to navigate many new situations. They can get help and support from a trusted confidant in dealing with both social- and age-related challenges such as going to college, getting a first job, or even getting married.

- **For the sibling, there is an opportunity to enjoy helping another person,** and we know from many studies, this results in greater maturity and increased tolerance of others.

Family Dynamics in Multigeneration AS

In some families, especially where there is AS in several generations, the family becomes guarded and sealed off from the world. In these cases, a "my tribe" (what one man with AS called it) mentality can occur—the idea that the only people who can be trusted are family members. The family wants to hide their issues; there may be unacceptable behavior taking place, and they begin to have secrets that must be guarded. The family does not want the rest of the world to know about their problems and difficulties in functioning, and the members band together in mutual distrust of the rest of the world.

This situation leads to four problems. First, having something to hide breeds feelings of distrust and introduces a bias against anyone who is an outsider, meaning not family. The distrustfulness all too often becomes a self-fulfilling prophecy as when, for example, the family with AS in their midst misinterprets the friendliness of others as nosiness and reacts negatively. The outsider feels rebuffed and will probably withdraw. The final step in this loop is the interpretation of the backing away as rejection. The AS family will feel justified in their distrust of the world, and their negative feelings about others will be reinforced.

The second problem is that the guardedness means the individual with AS will have limited opportunity to encounter many different kinds of people and is far less likely to gain important social skills.

The third problem is the person with AS will learn to depend on unconditional acceptance simply because he or she is one of the "tribe" or family.

The fourth problem is that there may be no expectations for the person with AS to learn appropriate limits for behavior because of poor personal boundaries in the family. To have personal boundaries means that the individual has a clear identity, a sense of who they are as a person, and a clear awareness of the limits that separate one individual from another. A person who has poor boundaries can't distinguish the differences between their own needs, feelings, opinions, and priorities and those of people around them. Having a good sense of our own boundaries makes us aware when someone is mistreating us, for example, by trying to push us into doing something we don't want to do or taking something that is ours without asking permission. Boundaries help us to have relationships as equals, where both parties' needs are equally valid. In some families, the person is not seen as an individual with his or her own needs and wants but is simply expected to go along with what the other person wants. This is what is meant by the term "enmeshed family" that is so often talked about in psychological problems. It is the job of the parent to help a child learn to develop personal boundaries as a part of establishing and maintaining mental health.

In some cases, if a family has a history of several generations of AS, it is very likely that the members of the family will not have good boundaries and will not be able to teach their children to have their own boundaries. The reason that families with several generations of AS have problems with boundaries is because one of the core impairments in people with AS is having trouble understanding that others have minds, feeling, needs, etc., of their own. As a result, they are likely to have little or no awareness that others' needs should be respected. In some rare cases, the lack of clear boundaries means that family members don't understand the idea of unacceptable behavior such as using a family member to get inappropriate needs met. These needs may include turning to a sibling or a child for the emotional needs that should be directed to a spouse or significant other. This use of a family member to get intimate emotional needs met (demands for an inappropriate level of emotional intimacy) has been called emotional incest. This lack of good boundaries can even sometimes lead to actual physical incest. In such a case, it is critically important to get professional intervention, and the parent and child may need to be physically separated.

What Are Ways to Improve Family Dynamics?

Family dynamics like these can be very hard to change, but if one family member seeks help or is referred for help because of some problem such as school performance, the cycle may be broken. Once the diagnosis of AS is made, a number of family difficulties will become understandable, and hopefully the family will get the help that is needed.

Friendship and AS

Friendships present an area of AS functioning that seems to vary widely, depending on the severity of the AS a person has, his or her personal history, and the experience the person has had with people outside the family. It also depends a lot on how much the adult with AS wants to have friends. A number of adults with AS seem to become less interested in friendships once they are working and/or married. These circumstances may provide all the social contact they want or need; and this is most often the case for those people who find it difficult to deal with many different people.

Maria's family had invited four of her classmates to spend a long weekend at their vacation home to celebrate Maria's twenty-first birthday. It was obvious that Maria was becoming more and more stressed. The pitch of her voice had gone up, and she kept echoing phrases that people were saying.

"Maria. Are you okay?" asked her mother, who had hoped Maria would enjoy having her friends join them in celebrating with her. Maria's parents have tried very hard to help her develop social skills and to make friends.

"I can't stand it when there are so many people around me. I wish they hadn't come. They stand too near me, and I can't stand to have them talking to me all the time. I wish they would just go home." The stress of a large volume of social interaction had become too much for Maria.

Some individuals with AS are more comfortable being in relationships with marginalized people. These relationships may be based on the feelings of sympathy mentioned in Chapter Seven, or marginalized people may seem simply less threatening or demanding.

For AS-NT couples, it is often the NT person (whether male or female) who will "manage" the friendships and facilitate the participation of the person with AS. Interestingly, however, in our experience, the decision of whom to include as friends is often made by the person with AS and quite consistently is based on some shared special interest.

How Can the Person with AS Manage Friendships?

It's important to keep in mind that friends are a key element in good support systems, and even if at times it seems like too much effort, it's very important to at least keep in touch by telephone or mail. It's also important to remember that friendships need to be mutual and that friends need to be listened to and supported in return.

On a lighter note...

Two friends meet in a card store at the mall.

"Why are you buying all those birthday cards, Naomi?"

"You won't believe this, but we were almost late for my sister's birthday celebration the other day. We were driving to the restaurant, and Jerry asked me the date. I said it was June 21st. He pulled into the next parking lot, and before I knew it, he was turned in the other direction. I asked him, "Where are we going? What's going on?"

"I've got to get a birthday card for Phyllis. It's her birthday on Monday!" was his reply.

"Who is Phyllis?" I asked him.

"My first secretary. You remember."

How could I have forgotten? She had been his secretary almost 25 years earlier! But I never have the chance to forget that he must send a birthday card to everyone he's ever known. He told me once he remembers every birth date he has ever heard. He is absolutely obsessive about sending a birthday card to everybody he has ever known. He told me that was his way to keep in touch with people he knows. He said people call him and tell him how wonderfully thoughtful he is. He loves it. So I thought, "I'll make it easier on myself. I'll make sure he has a whole stack of cards and stamps. No more detours or running late, I hope!"

Summing It All Up

In addition to parents, siblings, and friends, there are many other sources for support. Other sources people can turn to for help include religious figures such as ministers, priests, or rabbis. Members of the helping professions, such as psychologists, psychiatrists, or counselors, can, if they understand AS, provide helpful support also. Mentors of all sorts, such as coaches, colleagues, or a caring boss, are excellent resources for understanding situations and navigating them safely. What is important is to recognize the need for a broad-based support structure and figure out how to put it in place. Sometimes it helps to use the people who are already in place, such as parents or siblings, to help figure out who to add to the list and sometimes to help establish the relationship. We all need to know that there are people there for us. In the next chapter, we'll be talking about what's probably the most important source of support for most adults, AS or NT, and that is the support of a spouse.

CHAPTER NINE

How Marriage Is
Affected by AS

"I wasn't sure if I should marry Meg. We knew each other ever since grade school. Once we went out on a double date when we were in middle school and didn't like each other. In fact, we hated each other," said Mike.

Christine asked, "Hated each other? That's pretty strong."

Mike continued, "She thought she was smart, and she never stopped talking. She kept trying to decide what we should do like she thought she was in charge. Meg came from the richest family in town. She kept talking about people and whether they had money or not. Finally I said, 'I'm going home.' And then she started criticizing me, saying I had no manners."

"How did you two ever end up married?" asked Christine.

"A guy I knew from high school, Tom, was at Penn State with me. He was dating Meg's roommate Donna. Donna's parents wouldn't let her come up to Penn State alone, so Tom fixed it up for Meg and I to double date with him and Donna. That way the girls could come up together."

"That still doesn't explain why you married Meg," said Christine.

"Well, she really wanted to marry me, and college was almost over. So every one seemed to be settling down and getting married. I didn't have a job, and I didn't know what I wanted to do. She said if we got married, she would work and I could go to graduate school to study physics. I've been interested in physics ever since I was little—in fact, some people thought I was weird and called me 'the professor.' Anyway, the plan seemed to make sense, so we got married right after I graduated."

Mike and Christine had met at work. Mike's wife had just divorced him, and he was obsessed with the idea that he wanted to marry Christine. It was as if he was on a mission to marry again. Christine liked Mike, but in a lot of ways, he seemed different and sort of cold. He devoted almost all of his time to his research, and he wasn't very interested in socializing. His story about his marriage to Meg shocked her. How could you marry someone that you hadn't even liked? It didn't make sense to Christine, and she wasn't sure what to make of Mike. He was a really smart guy and always very polite in a stiff, formal way. But she found herself wondering who this man really was. Mike has not told Christine that he has AS. It's not clear that he agrees with the diagnosis.

For many years, little attention was paid to marriage in autistic spectrum disorders, mostly because it was believed that people on the autistic spectrum did not marry or have families. We now know better, and, in fact, several books have been published by couples where one or both partners have Asperger Syndrome (AS). Maxine Aston, a U.K. expert on counseling couples where AS is involved, has also written extensively about AS couples. This material gives us a good idea about some of the challenges faced by people with AS who do marry as well as some good strategies to help the couple make the marriage work. And no doubt, there are probably many couples affected by AS whose marriages work out successfully and who never come to the attention of professionals or the broader public.

The core difficulties of AS, however, frequently do present a challenge to working out a relationship as emotionally intimate and interdependent as marriage. The AS-related problems in communication, the difficulty in understanding another person's thoughts and feelings, the inflexibility, and the narrow and rigid interests all tend to interfere with the closeness, emotional intimacy, and support that most people seek in marriage. The chances of successfully working out these differences are much better if the diagnosis of AS has been made and accepted by the person with AS, and the couple has an understanding of what the presence of AS will mean to the relationship.

Choosing a Marriage Partner
We know that many people with autistic spectrum disorders do marry, and many of these marriages are probably to NTs. Some

have questioned why these unions happen. Some of the reasons we have heard and that have been written about make sense when you understand about AS. Many smart people are drawn like magnets to other bright people, and because many people with AS have very high IQs, they can be attractive partners. The person with AS also is likely to have in-depth knowledge about his or her special interest area, and this expertise can be very impressive.

Many people with AS, especially men, are quiet because they are somewhat guarded or do not enjoy talking. In fact, many women who have married a man with AS will say that, when she met him, he was a handsome, quiet stranger whom the woman thought she could help become more sociable. His quietness may also appear to be calmness, and for women who may have grown up with chaos and turmoil in their lives, this calm is very appealing.

The rigidity of AS thinking can come across as strength of character, and many men with AS do behave in honest, loyal ways. This can be extremely appealing to a woman who is looking for stability and commitment in life.

For men with AS, age does not seem to be a major consideration. A number of men with AS choose a partner who's considerably older than they are. This may be because many people with AS have little concern for social convention. Or it could be that the older person is someone the person with AS feels he or she can learn from or who will be more understanding. Another factor that in some cases influences the choice of a mate by a person with AS is the tendency to select a person who is marginal, such as someone with minority status or a physical problem.

Many women with AS are also not talkative, possibly for the same reasons as men with AS (guardedness or not liking to talk). They tend to be quite straightforward in their comments or when stating what they want or need. Women with AS are not usually interested in small talk and rarely engage in conversation about other people or emotions. These traits may be very appealing to some men or even come as a relief to men who are not comfortable with too much emotion. There is some information to suggest that women with AS may tend to chose as a partner a man who is much older or who may have health problems, perhaps feeling more comfortable with someone who may make fewer demands of them.

There is not a lot of information about marriages where both partners have AS, but having similar characteristics may lead to more understanding and less stress in the relationship.

Some common themes in AS-NT marriages

- Most people with AS will look for someone who is very competent in some way that complements their own abilities. Perhaps as a compensation for their own difficulties, many men with AS are drawn to someone with a great deal of social competence or a person who is very good at dealing with the problems of life.

- A number of AS men are drawn to NT women (and vice versa) who are more comfortable in the role of caretaker, rather than being in a more give-and-take partnership.

- There is a tendency for both the AS and NT partner to idealize the relationship. If people are not realistic about what human

232

relationships are all about, the disappointment that is a normal part of "the honeymoon being over" is often more severe. In a number of cases, the disillusionment has been extreme.

Like most courting couples, both NTs and those with AS tend to be on their best behavior during the earliest stages of the relationship, and it may be more difficult to see the signs of AS differences. If, however, you are familiar with the symptoms of AS, the differences can often be seen. In the story below of Harry and Carolyn, Harry's extreme interest in boating is an indication that he probably thinks in a different way from someone who is NT.

"Our invitation to the christening for Jane and Alex's new baby came today. It's a week from this Sunday. It'll be so nice to see the baby and to visit with family. It will give you a chance to meet my brother and his wife, too." Smiling, Carolyn handed the invitation to Harry.

"You know that we planned to spend weekends on the boat this summer. I told you I have work I want to do on the engine, and it needs some work done on the electronics," said Harry. "I wish you wouldn't plan something else every weekend. The summer will soon be over, and we won't have spent any time at all on the boat."

Carolyn looked surprised. "That's not true. We've been on the boat every weekend except for my uncle's funeral in June."

Harry was adamant that he was right, until Carolyn went to the calendar that they kept their schedules on. Sure enough, every weekend was noted "boating this weekend" except for the weekend of June 7, when "boating" was crossed out and "Uncle John's funeral" was filled in.

Harry did not say anything, but he became more quiet than usual and left early to return to his own apartment. He didn't answer his phone that evening, even though he had caller ID and knew it was Carolyn calling. Carolyn was upset. She had no idea what had gone wrong.

What Carolyn didn't know was that Harry's behavior was a part of his AS. It's difficult for people with AS to be thwarted when they want to do something that involves their special interest. Harry was obsessed with his boating, and it has been his special interest for many years. In addition, Harry, like many people with AS, does not enjoy socializing with people he doesn't know, so going to the christening does not appeal to him.

Carolyn made her point about how they had spent the summer weekends by bringing out their calendar. It showed that Harry was mistaken. Unfortunately, this only made the situation worse. Harry is better at dealing with facts than feelings, but in this case, the facts proved him to be wrong. And Harry, like many people with AS, has trouble ever being wrong.

AS-NT Marriages

There are people with AS who choose not to marry. Temple Grandin has commented publicly that the stress of marriage is something that she feels she does not want to undertake. Other people with AS struggle to manage their own lives, and marriage is not a consideration. In still other instances, the person with AS lacks the social skill to establish a relationship. But there are a number of AS-NT and AS-AS marriages, and while it is likely that many of these relationships work, there are a number that run into serious problems. As the stress of life begins to overshadow the idealization of the relationship, both parties begin to react to AS-NT difficulties. For the NT person, the lack of emotional responsiveness begins to feel like a rejection, and she begins to question the person with AS about what is happening. The person with AS, because of his problems with theory of mind, probably has no idea what she is talking about. He may become angry or even more withdrawn. This is likely because he interprets the questions as criticisms and because he wants to avoid conflict, sometimes at any cost. The NT partner does not understand this and, feeling lonely and frustrated, pursues even more, trying to establish some emotional connection. The response of the AS partner is to feel more pressured and to become even less available, often retreating to his special interest or even resorting to "stimming" to manage his stress.

Stimming is a repetitive behavior that, through regular repetition at times of stress, lowers the anxiety level of the person with AS. In young children with AS, it may involve a motor behavior like spinning in circles and flapping their hands, but as the person grows more mature, he or she likely substitutes a more socially acceptable behavior. One man with AS would spend hours playing solitaire on the computer, whereas a woman with AS would practice yoga headstands over and over. Both were using these repetitious behaviors to bring down their level of anxiety.

Marriage and Undiagnosed AS

If the diagnosis of AS has not been made, the AS pattern of difficulties, namely problems with understanding and expressing emotion and problems with communication, begins to take a toll on the relationship. In many cases, once the relationship has been established, the person with AS no longer feels that he must make the effort to maintain the relationship. The individual with AS will stop paying attention to his partner and will expect the NT spouse to act in the role of a caretaker, assuming responsibility for running the household. The special interests of the person with AS begin to take up most of his free time. The demands for routine and predictability that are an essential part of AS begin to take control of the couples' lives. AS begins to paralyze the relationship.

As the NT partner increases efforts to be close and to communicate, it leads to more intense negative emotion or withdrawal by the partner with AS. Anger and sadness swirl together, poisoning the atmosphere. And when the diagnosis of AS is not known, there is no explanation for what is going on. The AS partner becomes more stressed, controlling, or withdrawn, and the NT tries desperately to understand what is happening. It is at this point that the NT or the couple is likely to seek professional help. Unfortunately, far too many clinicians are unaware of AS. They resort to psychodynamic explanations, such as "the pursuer and the pursued," instead of helping the couple to understand that what they are dealing with is a difference in the way their brains function (and the two quite different cultures that exist as a result of that). In many cases, NTs are told that they are pursuing too hard and that they must change. The individuals with AS, because of the difficulty they have understanding others' minds and needs, will feel vindicated and will have increased resistance to change.

Sandy is at the end of her rope. Her husband's youngest brother Robert had once again behaved with absolutely no consideration for anyone. Showing up at ten o'clock at night, he had five college friends in tow instead of the two that she had expected. They had gone through the refrigerator and kitchen cabinets like a horde of locusts. She knew that the food she had bought for Thanksgiving dinner wasn't going to be nearly enough for three extra twenty-year-old guys.

Robert and his friends had stayed up all night watching videos. The sound from the TV was so loud, her bedroom floor vibrated. And now, at 4:30 in the afternoon, just as she was trying to finish the Thanksgiving dinner preparations, they were up and hungry, roaming in the kitchen. Robert was frying up a dozen eggs, making hamburgers, and opening baked beans; he had the entire kitchen in chaos. She went to search for Frank, her husband. Robert resented her and simply refused to respond to her, so there was no use trying to talk to him. She needed Frank's help if the rest of the family was to have any Thanksgiving dinner. She found Frank lying on the bed with his laptop open, once again playing a computer game. As she tried to explain what was going on, Frank became more agitated and accused her of not liking Robert and always criticizing him and his family. When Sandy tried to explain her side of the story,

Frank got up and walked outside. Dinner was a disaster. That night, Frank began sleeping in a guest bedroom; he refused to discuss what had happened, accusing Sandy of starting the problem and telling her she was crazy. How could a relationship that seemed so right go so wrong in such a short time?

Sandy had encountered some of the issues of AS that can be very hard on a marriage. Many people with AS have very serious problems dealing with conflict, and setting limits on a willful teenage sibling is most likely going to involve conflict. It's not clear that Frank understood the situation and how Robert bringing additional friends, unexpectedly during a holiday weekend, caused a lot of problems. It is difficult for someone with AS to see the big picture, and Frank couldn't grasp that having three extra people for five days would mean more work for Sandy, who also held down a full-time job.

Frank not acknowledging the inconsiderate behavior of the boys the night before made Sandy feel as though Frank had no concern for her and her well-being. The truth is, to deal with that situation would have probably meant another confrontation of which Frank wanted no part. And the final straw for Sandy, Robert arrogantly taking over the kitchen while she was trying to prepare a holiday meal for the rest of the family, simply didn't register with Frank. He was mind blind to Sandy's thoughts and feelings and felt that her demands were unreasonable. When she became upset, he bluntly called her crazy because it seemed irrational to Frank that she was upset by what was happening. Sandy had begun to notice that Frank often misinterpreted or got twisted in his mind things that happened when there was a lot going on or there was emotion involved. And always, he and his family were always right, and everyone else was wrong (remember the tribal mentality discussed in Chapter Eight?).

Sandy could not believe that Frank could be so callous and uncaring when she had made such an effort to make the holiday together special. She did not know that Frank was focused on his own need to avoid conflict and that he was not able, because of his AS, to understand the situation and to see the impact of Robert's self-centered behavior on his wife and the rest of the family.

Variations on these themes of the partner with AS not understanding the NTs distress and the NT feeling frustrated and unsupported get played out over and over in the misunderstandings in AS-NT relationships. Until there is a diagnosis, there is almost no way to work to resolve the misunderstandings. If, however, the condition of AS has been diagnosed and the diagnosis is accepted, then there are several steps to understanding that may help the relationship be more successful.

Building Understanding Between the AS and NT Worlds

- Having AS interferes with the ability to predict or understand the consequences of behavior on others. Frank did not understand the impact of Robert's behavior on Sandy. As a result, he saw her as irrational instead of recognizing how selfish and thoughtless Robert's behavior was.

- It is very important to most NTs, especially NT women, to have their partners understand them and their feelings. Recognizing and accepting that with an AS spouse this is not likely to happen, NT partners need to decide what is important to them. If they feel there are enough good things about the relationship and that they can find the support they need elsewhere, there is a good chance the relationship can work. It is not fair or realistic to expect the person with AS to be able to change enough to fully meet those needs.

• People with AS, but AS men in particular, may find conflict intolerable and often hear a difference of opinion, or an attempt to explain a different perspective on a situation, as conflict or criticism.

• The problems with boundaries that many people with AS frequently have means that any sort of criticism of members of their family of origin (unless for some reason they themselves dislike that family member) may be interpreted as criticism of them, and they will likely not be willing to tolerate it.

• Fundamental problems in communication are among the most important issues in an AS-NT relationship. Difficulty occurs with both speaking and hearing. Many men with AS simply cannot hear when a significant other discloses her emotions and feelings, especially if they are negative. Many men with AS will refuse to communicate at all if they are upset, although occasionally they will lose their temper and may lash out in a very hurtful way.

Being aware of these differences helps each party make sense of what is happening. Taking things personally will only make the situation worse. The AS and NT brains work differently, and it is useful for both the NT and the person with AS to develop an understanding of how those differences affect thinking and behavior.

What Is Necessary to Facilitate Change in an AS-NT Marriage?
- The difficulties people with AS tend to have in generalizing learning, changing behavior, and understanding others make it hard for them to alter their response and to change behavior. To do so requires a tremendous effort, and usually the person with AS has to have a real commitment to the relationship in order to make these changes possible.

- NT individuals may be more flexible and are usually more comfortable with change. For them, the decision must be, given what they know about AS and how it affects a relationship, are they willing to make a commitment?

How Can AS-NT Marriages Prosper?
To make an AS-NT marriage work, it is useful to have professional help—an impartial third party who can help the couple to untangle their interactions and tease out what role AS is playing. This will only work, however, if the therapist understands AS. The nature of AS means that the person with AS will not be able to see the impact of his behavior on his spouse; he will only see her reaction. As a result, he will tell the therapist the truth as he saw it, and he will probably try to invalidate his wife's version of

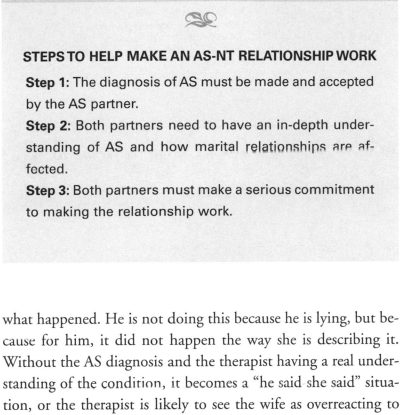

STEPS TO HELP MAKE AN AS-NT RELATIONSHIP WORK

Step 1: The diagnosis of AS must be made and accepted by the AS partner.

Step 2: Both partners need to have an in-depth understanding of AS and how marital relationships are affected.

Step 3: Both partners must make a serious commitment to making the relationship work.

what happened. He is not doing this because he is lying, but because for him, it did not happen the way she is describing it. Without the AS diagnosis and the therapist having a real understanding of the condition, it becomes a "he said she said" situation, or the therapist is likely to see the wife as overreacting to "normal male behavior." In these cases, which are far too common, the therapist fails both the AS and NT partner, because they are not getting the help needed to work out the relationship. And, in addition, the NT partner is twice wounded. The first wound to the NT is the therapist's failure to validate the wife's account of the situation and the hurt she experienced. The second wound is blaming the wife for the problems by saying she is overreacting.

242

"I have two chronic medical conditions that my doctors tell me are both stress-related. My rheumatoid arthritis has become, as you can see, so bad that I can hardly walk, and my hands can't hold a pen. I have a Ph.D. in microbiology, but I haven't been able to work in a laboratory for ten years because my hands are so crippled. I want desperately to leave my marriage, but I have no way to support or even care for myself. My husband is a good man—a kind man in many ways. He is a brilliant materials scientist with several patents. He tithes to our church and volunteers to deliver Meals on Wheels two Saturdays a month. But the stress of living with him is slowly killing me." The woman sitting in my office looked ten years older than the age listed on her medical insurance card.

Ellison, her husband who has AS, said, "I hope you can fix Mildred, doctor. She's been an invalid for years, and it is getting worse."

"I am not an invalid!" Mildred's sudden, sharp retort startled me. "You have been saying that for years. The truth is I am not an invalid! You have made me *invalid!* You have invalidated every word I've ever said when I try to explain to you my experience of what is happening. You are always right; I am always wrong. If I try to make my point by bringing up something you told me so you could see how the situation we are talking about is similar, you accuse me of being mean and using what you tell me against you. And you say that if I were truly kind, I would never do that. I am kind; I am just trying to get you to really see me and who I am and to see my side of what's happened. And every time I try to do that, you invalidate me. You make me *invalid*." Mildred suddenly stopped.

"See, Doctor. She's always accusing me of something or criticizing me. Other people think I am a kind man. I know because they tell me all the time. I hope you can fix her. Sometimes I think she is a mean person inside. I don't think I trust her anymore."

Mildred and Ellison were caught up in forces that neither one of them understood. They were two exceptionally smart people who didn't know how to bridge the gap in understanding between them. Their situation had some strengths with which to work because they were both very bright, well-educated people with minds trained to depend on logic and to think logically. They had many things in common. They were both trained as scientists, they shared strong religious values, and both were committed environmentalists. But the marriage, sadly, had a number of strikes against it that might prove fatal.

The threats to Mildred and Ellison's marriage
- Mildred was no longer emotionally committed to the marriage.
- Mildred was very angry that Ellison continually invalidated what she said.
- Ellison accepted no responsibility for problems in the marriage.
- Ellison had an unshakeable image of himself as good and kind.
- Ellison could not stand to be wrong.
- Ellison had made up his mind that it was Mildred who needed fixing—her thinking was not logical, and she was mean and not trustworthy.

Mildred was in a very difficult position. Her medical problems made her dependent, but the trauma of living with someone with undiagnosed AS had reached a point where it felt unbearable. It was not clear that Ellison would be willing, or even able, to hear a diagnosis of AS. He was extremely bright and very early in life had decided that he was a kind man because he engaged in certain "kind" behaviors. His self-image was based, to a great extent, on being smarter than other people in most instances and on always being right, and any suggestion that he might not be seeing or interpreting things accurately would probably be hard for him to accept. The only kind of information about himself that he felt comfortable hearing was validation of how he sees himself. He had repeated the statement, "Other people think I am a kind man. I know because they tell me," several times during the session.

When Mildred challenges his self-perception by trying to talk about her experience, he believes she is just attacking or criticizing him. His need to see himself as kind and never wrong makes him hypersensitive to criticism. If, in an attempt to get him to understand what she is trying to tell him, Mildred repeats something he has told her about himself, he feels betrayed and that she is being mean and deliberately hurting him.

If Ellison accepted what Mildred was saying, he would have to change the image he has of himself, which is difficult for all of us. But for someone with AS who lacks cognitive flexibility, changing their self-image it is extremely difficult or sometimes impossible. The black and white tendency in AS thinking can translate to something being "all good" or "all bad," and with

Ellison's hypersensitivity to criticism, the possibility of being "all bad," when his current self-image is "all good," would likely be devastating. By the same token, to be diagnosed as having AS, a condition that means there is a neurological difference in his mind, would probably be too threatening for Ellison, who values his thinking and logic very highly, to bear.

If Mildred begins to understand that Ellison has AS and the way Ellison's mind works as a result of it, she may be able to "validate" herself. She can begin to understand why things occur between them as they do and to change her expectations of their relationship. In this case, they may be able to redefine the relationship in a way that they can continue to be together, although living with little emotional closeness.

Making Accommodations for AS-NT Relationships

Realistically, for an AS-NT marriage to work, it's likely that the NT will have to make more accommodations than the person with AS, even if the partner with AS accepts the diagnosis and makes every effort to learn different ways of behaving. Many NTs, mostly women, have told us that the difference in expectations is unfair; why should they make all the accommodations? The issue is not a matter of fairness. AS means that the individual's brain has developed differently than the brain of someone who is NT. There is no known way to change that difference. As a result of the difference, AS brains operate differently from NT brains, and some activities NT brains do automatically (for example, interpreting nonverbal communication) must be done by a different part of the AS brain, and usually require a great deal of effort.

Even when the person with AS is trying very hard to "figure things out," there is a strong likelihood, as we saw in the section on shy gorillas in Chapter Eight, that their conclusion will be wrong. There is too much nonverbal information in the NT world that a person with AS will not understand or will not understand correctly. To expect the person with AS to be able to logically work his or her way through the subtle, complex, sometimes irrational processes of the NT world is a bit like thinking that, if you can hum along to a tune, you should be able to compose a symphony like Beethoven's Fifth. Some amount of the NT world will probably always be invisible to a person with AS. If the focus in the relationship can be shifted from what is not there or what is wrong to what is good, the strengths of AS can be valued. And if people with AS can realize that as a result of the differences in the way their brain works, their perception of themselves may not be accurate and they may be prone to misunderstanding situations and misreading their spouse's intentions in discussions, it may be possible for the couple to find a way to manage their relationship.

Ways to Improve an AS-NT Marriage

• For the NT, shift your focus from what you are not getting from your AS partner to see and value the strengths he or she brings to the relationship.

• For the AS person, reconsider your perception of yourself and accept that, because of the differences in the way your brain works, what your partner is telling you about your role in problems is probably right.

- For both NTs and individuals with AS, try to listen to one another in a nondefensive way. Ask for clarification of things you don't understand in a simple, respectful, low-key way—and you might just improve communication!

Other Aspects of Marriage

Our focus until now has been on how the differences in AS-NT thinking and communications can interfere with AS-NT couples understanding of one another. But there are many other dimensions to marriage. Let's first look at the impact of AS on sexuality.

Sexuality

As we have already noted, there's not a lot of research about AS in adults, including AS and sexuality. However, both Maxine Aston, the U.K. couples' counselor, and Dr. Isabelle Henault, a Canadian AS researcher, have done some research that makes it clear that people with AS do have an interest in sexual matters and, not surprisingly, that AS can and may play a role in how these sexual interests are played out. As is the case with NTs, many of the sexual issues in AS-NT relationships are because of psychological or emotional difficulties the couple is having. There are several exceptions to this. One exception involves the problems with hypersensitivity some people with AS experience. This reaction may be to smell, touch, or textures such as nightwear or bed coverings. Fortunately, in many cases, these problems can be managed if they can be identified. Changing to a comfortable fabric for sheets or nightwear or using certain products, such as face cream without fragrance, may reduce the problem. It's helpful for the couple to address these issues as soon as they occur to prevent further problems from developing in the relationship. A second exception involves the AS bias toward not having to deal with someone else's feelings or needs. In this case, some people with AS prefer masturbation to intercourse because it is does not involve all the complication of having to be concerned with someone else's needs.

A Lack of Sexual Activity in Marriage
There are other sources of sexual problems. Ms. Aston reports, in her book *Aspergers in Love,* that in as many as 50 percent of her research sample of AS-NT marriages where the AS partner is male, there has been no sex in the marriage for a number of years. This finding is in agreement with a lot of clinical evidence.

"We haven't had sex for two years now, and we've only been married for three. When we did have sexual relations, I had to be the one to initiate it. I didn't know if Paul really wanted to make love or if he was just doing it to please me. It makes me feel so unattractive, like I am not desirable,' said MaryAnn.

"It's not that," Paul said. "I just can never tell if you want to have sex or just snuggle. I never seem to get it right, and it just doesn't seem worth the bother. You know it doesn't have to be such a big deal. People can satisfy themselves. It's not like you need to have some skill, like when you are fixing a car."

Paul and MaryAnn's story contains some of the sexual problems that come up in AS-NT marriages. Paul has come to the conclusion that there is too much to worry about if he has sex with MaryAnn. With his AS-related problems with understanding nonverbal communications, it is not surprising that he has trouble, or perhaps can't even read at all, subtle nonverbal cues that are so much a part of sexual relationships. If we add to this the difficulty people with AS have in understanding the timing of interpersonal relationships and their difficulty figuring out the pace of things (when it is their turn to "do something"?), sexual interactions can become loaded with anxiety. Is he picking the right behavior for the right time? Is he initiating intimate relations when what she wants is to cuddle? Paul's comments about people satisfying themselves suggest that he has decided that it is much simpler to masturbate to meet his sexual needs.

MaryAnn voices what is probably the most common complaint heard from NT women in AS-NT relationship. MaryAnn wants not only a sexual relationship but one that meets her emotional needs of feeling wanted and loved.

If there are difficulties with the sexual part of a relationship, feelings of anxiety, frustration, and disappointment can occur, and these feelings can spill over into other areas of a relationship that may already be troubled.

Impotence

Impotence, the inability to achieve an erection, is one of the more commonly cited problems in AS-NT relationships. There are many causes of impotence, and the possibility of impotence being a physical problem should be assessed and ruled out. But more frequently, the problem behind the impotence is a psychological one. In many cases, the man may not truly be impotent; he may prefer the more solitary experience of masturbation, where he has complete control and doesn't have to worry about pleasing his partner. Or the issue may be unresolved anger directed toward his partner. As mentioned before, men with AS tend to avoid conflict and are not willing to address what is bothering them with their partner. Instead, he may withdraw, verbally, physically, and sexually, to get his message across to her that he is angry and resort to masturbation to meet his physical needs. This passive-aggressive behavior is hurtful; the spouse usually has no idea of what is wrong, and the husband refuses to communicate so she can't find out why he is upset. When this behavior goes on too long or happens too often, the partner suffers emotional abuse. Furthermore, once a man with AS has begun masturbating, as with many AS habits, it becomes a habit that is very hard to break. As a result, one more channel of possible communication is closed.

Premature Ejaculation and Retarded Ejaculation
Premature ejaculation is often associated in all men with worry or anxiety about performance—a state of mind that is fairly common in people with AS. The situation may be compounded by the difficulty many people with AS have in being in touch with the state of their mind and body; this may mean that the man with AS will not himself understand when he is about to have an orgasm.

Retarded ejaculation is an issue of control and being able to let go. If the man with AS is anxious, in some cases, rather than lose control and ejaculate prematurely, he will become so focused on control that he is not able to stop worrying long enough to release and voluntarily ejaculate.

Even though sex may not be high on the agenda in an AS-NT relationship, sexual problems still take a toll. Because of all the other fragile aspects of an AS-NT relationship, sexual problems may be especially damaging to both partners and therefore may be damaging to the survival of the relationship.

Sexuality in Women with AS

Sexuality seems to be less complicated for women with AS, and it is often described by them as an uncomplicated source of pleasure. One young woman with diagnosed AS reported that when she turned fourteen, she decided to sleep with the boy she was seeing because "boys like girls who are willing to have sex." Her mother found out that she planned to sleep with her boyfriend and took her for birth control pills. "It was good because I didn't have to worry about getting pregnant. I like sex, and I am comfortable sleeping with the man I'm dating."

It is a great concern that neither mother nor daughter seemed to be thinking about or making sure that the daughter took precautions to prevent sexually transmitted diseases. The AS difficulty with seeing the big picture may mean she didn't really understand the risk. This same young woman with AS did not see anything wrong with having sex with men outside her marriage. When asked about whether she was being fair to her husband, who was almost twenty years older than she was, she replied that since she didn't have sex with him because he was sick, and he didn't ask if she was having sex with anyone else, as far as she could see, there was no problem with it.

On a positive note, some AS-NT couples reported no problems with their sex life. In fact, these couples said the simple physical quality of the act seemed the simplest, easiest way to communicate loving feelings.

Problems with sexuality in a marriage tend to reflect problems that exist more broadly in the relationship, and these issues can be very difficult to untangle and resolve. For many couples, the sensitivity of the issue makes it even more difficult to discuss and resolve. For the AS-NT couple, where communication will probably be more difficult because of the impact of AS, it may be very difficult to discuss sexual problems without professional help from a counselor who understands AS.

Fidelity

Georgia was stunned. "You have a girlfriend? What are you saying? This can't be true! I don't believe it!"

"You've been traveling a lot. You know that I don't like to be alone. The kids are married now and have their own families. I just want to be happy, and I think I will be with Lorraine. She's lonely and told me that all she wants is to be with me. You are always busy," David said.

"But you know I travel for work because I have to. I've asked you to come with me," said Georgia. "You never want to. What could I do?"

Based on the information we have, the rate of infidelity is relatively low in AS men, and most AS men remain faithful to their partner. When men with AS do go outside their primary relationship, it is usually because someone else made them feel special at a time when they felt their partner was not paying them the kind of attention they wanted or if they had decided that they no longer liked their spouse.

The other reason cited by AS men who had affairs was that the women had some characteristic they were very drawn to, such as long dark hair or a special fragrance. Often, once an AS man starts down the road of infidelity, it is likely to become a pattern, as is the case with so many other AS behaviors.

The resolution of an affair depends mostly on the people involved and how far the affair has gone. As noted though, once people with AS establish a pattern, whether it is having affairs or any other behavior pattern, it is very hard for them to change it. With the differences in AS thinking and way of relating making the situation more complex, the best chance for a reasonable outcome is to seek counseling with a competent, knowledgeable counselor who understands AS.

Jealousy

Although not much has been written about it, some men and women with AS can and do sometimes suffer from intense jealousy. A woman with AS told her husband that if he ever looked at someone else, she would divorce him and make sure he had no contact with their child. A man with AS once said he thought he could forgive his partner for having been in a relationship before they met, but that he could never forget it. When he was questioned why he felt so strongly about this, since he and his wife didn't even know each other at the time she was with the other man, he seemed at a loss as to why he felt this way. He was a very bright man and a logical thinker. After giving the question some thought, the best explanation he could come up with was that he "just wished she hadn't done it, that's all." He continued to have feelings of jealousy about her even after their relationship ended.

Children

Parenting is another area of AS-NT marriages for which little information is known. But as one computer scientist who describes himself as having AS says, "We know AS is genetic, so some people with AS must be parents!" And as mentioned in Chapter Two, a number of adults have self-diagnosed or sought out a diagnosis of AS after hearing the symptoms when their child was diagnosed with AS. These adults recognized the symptoms in themselves or their spouse.

Having a child introduces a lot of change for any couple, and it is no different when one or both parents have AS. Change is almost always difficult for people with AS to manage, and the disruption can be substantial. One woman with AS had settled into marriage fairly easily. She did not need to worry financially. Her husband earned a good income and was a very generous person. But the birth of their first child, which was a planned pregnancy, was much more responsibility than she had understood (remember, people with AS often have a lot of difficulty anticipating outcomes). Her husband had to take on many of the responsibilities for running the household and caring for the child. The wife seemed to almost be in a sort of psychological shock and repeatedly said, "What about me? When can I start going out with the girls and having a drink or lunch?" It was very clear that she was struggling to understand that the child's needs had to take priority. The difficulty people with AS have understanding that others' minds and needs may be different from their own can sometimes result in the child not getting the correct care. In one case, the child's pediatrician had to intervene because the AS mother had limited the child's diet to pasta because that was all she, the mother, ate.

If both partners want the child, they are usually able to work out ways to manage, although the problems with mind blindness that are a part of AS may make it hard or not possible for the parent with AS to understand the child's needs and how to respond. One family managed this by setting up a schedule that spelled out what needed to be done for the child at what time. Such a system works well when the child is an infant but is not as useful as the child grows older. As the child matures, there is a greater need for flexibility, taking into account the child's individuality. It's helpful at that time for the NT parent to assume a more directive and active role.

Guarding the Child's Well-Being
The non-AS parent must be watchful when the child is not yet able to talk or is not able to tell people what is wrong. If something unusual happens, for example, if the young child develops an earache or toothache, the parent with AS, because of his or

her problems with understanding nonverbal communication, may not understand or may not notice the child's pain. The non-AS parent must remain vigilant to make sure the child is safe and well cared for.

If the Child Has AS
In situations where the child has AS, and either one or both parents have AS, parents often recognize their own behavior in the child. As a result, parents will find it easier to understand the child, and there will be less stress and tension in the family.

Considerations Before Having Children
The decision to have a child should be mutual and well discussed before commitments are made. It's a good idea for both parties to spend time with a family member who has children and to participate in the care of the children. Spending time with others' children makes what it means to have a child a lot more real. Each person in the relationship should be encouraged to discuss their roles in raising the child.

Children, AS, and Divorce
It is critically important to note that the AS parent does not intentionally not take care of the child, but rather that a person with AS does not have the intuitive abilities of a parent who is NT. This is in addition to the problems people with AS have in predicting outcomes, which at times means a parent with AS will perhaps not be able to see the impact of their behavior on the child, such as leaving a sleeping child home alone. These AS-related problems

can put the child at risk. This aspect of AS parenting presents a serious issue in the case of divorce. The parent with AS may fight for custody of the child or children for many reasons, as is the case in NT divorces. They may feel they are the better parent, or it may be a way to punish the other parent for leaving the relationship. No matter what the reason, the issue of custody will likely present a cause for serious concern on the part of the NT spouse. They will be aware of the problems with communication, the lack of empathy, and the problems of judgment that result from AS and have grave concerns about the safety and well-being of the child being left in the sole care of the parent with AS. But because AS is not well known or understood, the NT parent's concern about the child's welfare may not be taken seriously by the court. In many cases, the parent with AS may appear very high functioning and can be successful in a highly respected profession such as medicine or teaching. Further, because many high-functioning people with AS have learned to compensate for their AS-related problems when it is important to them to do so, they will make the effort to appear very competent. As a result, the court may be quite impressed with the individual—he is smart, successful, and seems to manage very well. There is no reason for the court to question the person's abilities to parent.

The problem is this: Compensating takes a great deal of effort, and a person with AS cannot sustain this effort all the time. In addition, the fundamental differences in functioning that are core to AS do not change. Unless there has been a diagnosis of AS made and the court is knowledgeable about AS, the court may be misled and judge the non-AS parent's concerns as attempts on the part of one parent seeking custody to discredit the other parent. In an AS-NT custody battle, which in some cases will be highly conflicted, the AS version of the family story will likely be inaccurate as a result of the AS problem with theory of mind. If the court does not understand AS, the court will see that version as being as credible as the version of the NT parent and will make its decision accordingly. As a result, the children may be unintentionally put at risk.

There is a major effort underway in the Canadian and U.K. courts to help judges become more knowledgeable about AS, the differences in thinking that it causes, and the possible consequences to all parties. There is a need for U.S. judges to become more aware of the syndrome to protect the welfare of children.

Finances

In marriages where AS is present, like all marriages, managing finances reflects a number of things: the knowledge and experience of the person managing the money, the resources the couple has, and their value system. Some people with AS are good at managing money, while others are described by the NT spouse as "not using common sense." One of the more frequently reported problems involving money in AS-NT marriages involves the breadwinner (most often the husband) using money to exert control of the family. He may insist that he must approve every purchase or he may dole out too little money to meet the family's basic needs, and the family ends up with a standard of living lower than their income level would suggest. In other cases, the partner with AS may spend excessive, even extravagant, amounts of money on his or her special interest, even if it means sacrifices have to be made by the rest of the family. Sometimes a person with AS will use money to "even a score" if he or she is angry with a spouse. People with AS usually cannot tolerate conflict and will not talk about the issue directly, and so they may find controlling money a satisfactory way to express their displeasure. Here is Deane and Andrew's story.

"We have almost seventy-five thousand dollars in credit card debt. I'm frantic. I'm afraid to answer the phone; it's always a collection agency. I had no idea that Andrew had run up all these bills. By the time we pay the monthly minimum, we hardly have enough to live on," Deane said.

"You spend money on whatever you want. You bought Jason [a grandchild] that little league outfit," responded Andrew.

"That was his birthday gift from both of us. We talked about it."

As the conversation continued, it became clear that money had become a battleground for this AS-NT couple. Andrew's AS thinking meant that it was hard for him to understand others' needs, and he felt, "I earn the money and I should decide how it is spent." Deana protested he had wanted her to stay at home and raise their family and that even the law recognized a wife's contribution had financial value.

"That's right," said Andrew, "And the law says that if the husband dies, the wife is responsible for his debt. My company has a seventy-five thousand dollar death benefit policy on me. It is money I've earned working there all these years. So I'm spending it while I can enjoy it."

Andrew, who is an extremely smart man, had figured out a way to keep in control of the couple's finances even after death. He kept his credit card debt equal to the amount of money his insurance policy would pay when he died. Many people with AS have very strong ideas about justice and injustice. Andrew felt it was unfair of Deane to spend money he earned, unless he had approved of what was being bought.

Many people with AS are very generous, and in some cases, this generosity can lead to financial problems and marital stress. One man with AS wanted very much to be liked. He found out when he was quite young that giving gifts resulted in positive responses, and people seeing him as a "really nice guy." His wife became very hurt and angry when she found out that the money she had saved to buy airline tickets for a long-awaited trip to the Caribbean was missing from their account. Asked what he knew about it, her husband replied that one of the cleaning people in his building hadn't been to her home to Jamaica for almost fifteen years. Since the money was earmarked for airline tickets anyway, he decided to surprise the cleaner with an airline gift certificate to take the trip. While his wife appreciated his generosity, this went too far for her! She was concerned because not only did her husband not take her feelings into account, his attitude toward money could cause problems with their future financial security.

What Are Ways Couples Can Handle Their Finances?
A number of AS-NT couples have decided that the NT partner will handle their money. Several of these couples have a rule that

any expense over some set limit will be discussed. This arrangement is often quite satisfactory to both partners. The NT will feel more confident about the finances, and the person with AS is relieved to have one less responsibility. In all cases, it's important that early on in the relationship, before behavior patterns are established, the couple should decide how finances will be handled. If that has not happened, a reliable financial advisor can give expert input to sort out finances and get the couple on the right track. In general, people with AS have a great deal of respect for expertise and are usually willing to listen to advice from an expert.

Summing It All Up

The impact of AS on a marriage is substantial and can cause a great deal of pain in many cases if the condition is not understood. If both partners have AS, understanding one another and common needs may make the relationship less stressful. If, however, the match involves an NT partner, the differences in the way someone with AS thinks and communicates may be devastating to the relationship. In fact, a name has been given to the condition of an NT spouse living with (usually unrecognized) AS—the Cassandra phenomenon. Cassandra was a character in Homer's Odyssey. The god Apollo fell in love with Cassandra and gave her the power to foretell the future. Cassandra refused his love, and although he could not take back the gift of prophecy, he put a curse on Cassandra that no one would believe her prophecies.

An NT partner living with a partner with undiagnosed or unacknowledged AS knows that something is wrong in the relationship. Not knowing about AS and the role it is playing in the relationship, she cannot explain why there are so many problems, but she knows the problems keep continuing to happen. She turns to others for validation and support or help in understanding. But because others usually only see the partner on his best behavior, her problems and her predictions about future problems are not believed.

Many of the differences that result from having AS can be very subtle, especially in high-functioning individuals. What's more, the person with AS will often put a great deal of effort into functioning well in public but will not be able or willing to function at that level at home. This situation leaves the people who know the couple with the impression that there is no problem, or if there is one, it's the NT's problem. As a result, when the non-AS spouse tries to get support and help for the many painful misunderstandings that occur, neither her spouse (whose AS means he will not be able to see his role in the problem) nor others will believe her, or they will insist that the problem is hers because she is too emotional or too sensitive and is overreacting. As a result, the NT spouse is greatly stressed and can develop depression or stress-related physical problems.

Few situations are insoluble, and if the AS has been diagnosed and acknowledged, and both partners are committed, it is possible that the couple will be able to work it out and stay in the relationship. The challenges are substantial and should not be undertaken lightly. In many cases, there will be a need for professional help to educate both partners about the nature of AS and what that means in day-to-day living. That is what we have attempted to do in this book.

CHAPTER TEN

Finding the Right Job:
The All-Important Career Choice

Keith's Story

"I started working in the computer lab while I was still an undergraduate. I was studying electrical engineering, but some of the stuff was really boring. What I really liked was seeing how far you could push the envelope with computers. If one computer was good, maybe two would be better. One of my professors was really interested in what I was doing. He got me interested in stuff the National Oceanographic Institute was doing with parallel computing. Some of the other guys from school heard about what I was doing at the lab, so I showed them how to set up the network. After I finished my masters, I didn't know what I wanted to do, so that same professor suggested I stay on and teach. So I did for a couple of years, and then he said while I was there, maybe I should get my doctorate. So I did. I stayed on after that for a while, but some stuff

happened in my life, and I got an offer to work at NSI (the National Science Institute). The rest is history. Here I am. I have a connection at my apartment to get to the computer at work, so I can work whenever I want to. In fact, I'm working on a new idea for using the Net. I don't want to talk about it, because I want to do it first."

Amy's Story

"Our oldest daughter, Amy, is a very special, very smart woman. She showed so much promise, but things never went right for her. She would do brilliantly in one class, amaze her teachers with her knowledge and understanding, and then barely get through some other subject. If she didn't like the subject, it seemed impossible to get her to do the work. We were so frustrated. One day, I sat her down and said, 'You will do what your teachers tell you to do. That is the rule. Don't ever break it.' I know it sounds strange, but it worked. She got mad and complained, but she did it.

She used to have fights with teachers in high school and with her college professors. If she thought she was right (and by darn, she usually was), she wouldn't back down. Lots of times, she would spend days searching for proof that she was right and knew what she was talking about.

Amy was very good in biology and took graduate-level courses while she was still an undergraduate. She wanted to be a veterinarian, and I think she would have been a good one. She loves animals. To tell the truth, she likes animals probably more than she likes people. She was always a loner. She had trouble keeping friends because things always had to be her way. We just couldn't figure out what was wrong and why she had such a hard time. I wish we'd known then that her problem is AS. Maybe we could have done things differently. She saw a lot of professionals. If I had all the money we spent on psychiatrists, I would retire, instead of still doing surgery at age sixty-nine. She's had almost every diagnosis in the book. I don't think anyone really knew what was wrong with her. My wife and I, especially my wife, worry to this day about what we may have done or didn't do to have her life turn out this way. It's hard for me to believe it, but Amy is now forty-three years old."

"What is she doing now?" I asked.

"She is living with a seventy-year-old man—a man a year older than I am—and grooming dogs at some dog hospital. What a terrible waste of so much promise. I don't know what we did wrong."

Sigmund Freud once summed up successful psychoanalysis as making it possible for the patient "to be able to love and to work." Much of what we've talked about so far could be said to focus on the world of "love," meaning the impact of Asperger Syndrome (AS) on relationships. As you can see from the opening stories, we are now turning to the world of work.

When it comes to AS and the world of work, as the two stories above show, there is a lot of variability in whether or not people with AS are able to get work that is meaningful to them and that allows them to use their talent to the fullest. For some individuals with AS, their passion about their special interest can, with thought and often guidance, result in remarkable success. In the first story, Keith's fascination with computers and his wish to push the power of computing to its limits led to his initial success. His professor, noting the success, took steps to encourage him to make the most of his talent, and to quote Keith, "The rest is history." For this young man, a number of forces came together that worked in his favor. Let's review these attributes that helped make his career successful.

- **A "special interest" that has vocational opportunities**
  Keith's choice, computer science, is a growing field that offers job opportunities.

- **"Islets of ability," the specialized abilities often seen in AS (see Chapter Five)**
  Keith's competence at logical, sequential thinking and an interest in mathematics meant that he would be good at his special interest.

- **Some ability to work with others**
  Being the expert, Keith felt comfortable because his skills were respected, and he was able work with the other students.

- **A good person-environment match**
  The world of computer research tends to be tolerant of brilliant loners and of eccentricities. Good interpersonal interactions or social skills are not always required.

- **A supportive, experienced mentor**
  Keith's professor respected students' abilities and had a knack
  for suggesting well-timed next steps.

It goes without saying that not all young people with AS
have things work out as well as they did for Keith. Amy's story
(as told by her father in a therapy session) suggests that she
functioned best in situations where there were boundaries and
clear rules. When Amy was told by her father that she must do
what her teachers told her to and that it was a rule, she then understood what was required of her and did it. Most people with
AS have respect for rules, and when Amy was given a rule for
how she was to behave, although she was not happy about it,
she followed it. Sadly for Amy, in the U.S. world of teens and
mental health, not to mention most school settings, there is
more emphasis on self-expression than on limits and rules.
Without a set of clear guidelines and instruction about what she
could and couldn't do, Amy lost her way, and she regularly got
sidetracked and caught up in efforts to prove she was right. In
most instances, this was a waste of time and took her away from
focusing on what she needed to do to accomplish her goal of
becoming a veterinarian. Not only that, but her behavior put
her at odds with her teachers and professors who did not understand that many of Amy's more problematic behaviors were a
result of her having AS. As a result, these teachers were probably not inclined to go out of their way to help her. Although her
parents recognized that Amy had a problem, their search for
help for their daughter was not successful. Unfortunately, the

true nature of Amy's problem, AS, was not recognized in the U.S. until 1994.

Amy did have a special interest, biology, and her academic performance in that subject suggests that she had considerable ability in that area. Her career goal, veterinary medicine, would have been compatible with her interest and ability. The difference between Keith's and Amy's career path was that Keith's interest had direct, early application, and he was able to "grow into" his current position. In Amy's situation, the way academia is set up meant that she had to spend a number of years studying things for which she probably didn't have a natural ability. And because of her AS, if a subject didn't interest her, Amy was not inclined to work at it. She also faced a series of hurdles that involved the need for communication (getting professors to understand what she needed and how her cognitive problems made certain academic requirements difficult for her to fulfill). Many of the interpersonal activities that were required of Amy to successfully navigate the world of academia (working with professors, guidance counselors, and admissions officers) were ones in which, as a result of AS, she lacked competence. Amy's lack of social competence and the lack of structure (for example, rules) in her life meant that she was denied the opportunity to use her considerable talents in a role that would have provided her much respect and opportunities for growth.

Social Competence in the Workplace

Many people with AS question whether all the emphasis on social competence is necessary or is just an attempt by the

NT-dominated society to impose its standards on the rest of the world. We believe there are two very important answers to that question. The first has to do with the emotional well-being of the person with AS. Most people with AS are lonely and are not often loners by choice. If you look closely at the depression and negativity that is associated with AS in adolescence and adulthood, you see that it is most often a result of the recognition by the person with AS that he or she can't establish or keep relationships. The second response as to why it is important to learn to socialize is that, in today's age, "knowledge work" takes precedence over manual labor. Most jobs involving knowledge work also involve working with, or as a part of, a team. Interpersonal skill is a valued commodity in our society, and to even get the chance to work, most people must go through an interview process that requires and assesses the person's "people skills." It's for these reasons that it is important for people with AS to make an effort to develop social competence.

If individuals with AS lack the social skills to manage the job interview process successfully and fail to get a job they are otherwise qualified for, they may turn to employment that does not suit them. It may be manual labor, where AS-related coordination problems will likely hinder adequate job performance, or a job even less suited to an AS temperament, such as doing telephone sales, a job that requires unrelenting contact with many different people. This kind of job not only requires constant contact with people, by itself a source of difficulty for people with AS, but it also means tolerating and coping with hostility from people who resent the intrusion of an unsolicited sales call. Most people with AS have problems dealing with anger and conflict, and as a result, a job like this would be extremely stressful. It's likely the person with AS would fail to perform adequately in this job or would not be able to tolerate the stress. Either way, the person would lose the job, failing once again. This process of rejection, trying at inappropriate work, and the resulting failure further undermines the individual's self-esteem and quite often leads to despondency or depression.

How Can an Adult with AS Cope in the Workplace?

There is unfortunately a lack of resources for social-skill training for adults with AS, and the resources that exist do not target individuals who are most able or who are high functioning. What's more, for many of these high-functioning people with AS, their problems are masked by their compensating skills, and their difficulties are not recognized.

There are ways to help, however. Many able people with AS resort to the behavior that has helped them cope for much of their life. They will identify high-functioning people and observe their behaviors. With a lot of effort, they will translate those behaviors into a form that will work for them. These models may be a parent or other family member (siblings are a frequent choice) or a trusted mentor. There are also professionals who can help the individual develop better ways to relate to other people at work, such as therapists who understand AS. Employment counselors can provide a script for a job interview and the opportunity to rehearse the script over and over again. If people with AS are already employed but wish to be promoted, they can seek out organizational consultants who do personal coaching designed to help people improve their social and communication skills to better position themselves for promotions. This is also the stage of life when many people seek out a partner either to live with or to marry. A number of people with AS choose someone they feel is competent and who can help them to be successful in the workplace by helping them to understand workplace politics or give them advice on organizing work.

Choosing a Career

Just as is the case with NTs, people with AS will want to choose a career that interests them or at which they are likely to be successful. We talked before about using special interests as an important way to define a career path. But if the special interest is something that does not translate well into a career path, such as knowing the name of the special effects man in every film ever made (although that information might come in handy on a game show!), a good alternative choice involves areas where the person with AS has natural abilities.

"I got a job. I'm going to work in the back office at Charles Schwab. I start right after I graduate in May," Gordon told his cousin Marc.

"Wow, I thought you were going to graduate school to study speech therapy." Marc was surprised at this turn of events. He knew that Gordon had started college with a goal of getting a doctorate in microbiology. He had spent long hours in

272

high school trying to master biology. When Gordon began college, the courses in organic chemistry were so difficult that he
decided to drop them. He had taken some business courses to
fill in his schedule, and he was graduating on time.

"What made you decide to apply to Schwab?"

"When I took accounting, I found it was really easy and that
I was really good at it. I won't have to work twenty-four hours
a day, and I'll be making good money. Who knows, maybe I'll
be president of Schwab one day!"

Marc, smiling, said, "Could be!" He knew that Gordon set
unusually high goals for himself.

Although Gordon started with a goal of studying microbiology, a natural extension of the "bugs" that had fascinated him as
a child, his experience in high school and then at college helped
him to understand that it would be very difficult for him to master some of the advanced courses he would need, such as organic
chemistry. With support from his family (who understood a lot
about AS because Gordon had been diagnosed several years ago),
he began to realign his studies with his strongest skills. He had a
real knack for working with numbers and figured out that he
could have a career doing something for which he was well suited.

How Can the Person with AS Choose the Right Career Path?
Think about things that you do well, and let those skills help
guide your career choice. It will really improve your chances of
being successful! Remember the following points in finding the
right job for you:

• Look for work that matches your interests, skills, and abilities.
• Make sure you try to develop your social competence. Strong social competence will help open the door to opportunity.

Summing It All Up

People with AS have different interests, different talents, and different levels of ability. There is no one piece of career advice that applies to all people. Some people with AS will have no difficulty finding a career with which they are satisfied and where they will stay for their entire work life. Others will need to try several different lines of work before they find something suitable. Still others may lose a series of jobs while they are learning the interpersonal skills that will make it possible for them to stay employed. There are some individuals with AS who need assistance from families and/or agencies to find work that fits their abilities.

Unfortunately, unlike countries like the U.K., the U.S. at this time does not have organizations that are able to help individuals with AS who need help finding employment. Hopefully, as AS becomes better known and understood in the U.S., these resources will be put in place.

Conclusion

The Blanket
For most of my life
I've been wrapped in a blanket

Whilst under it
I am unable to interact
Stuck with super glued outlooks
And thought patterns that circle
Over and over the same repeating facts.
Under this blanket
My movements lack the motors of response
And idiosyncratic gestures remain reclusive
Hidden under the thick blanket
Of behaviors often seen as illusive.
Watching the purple flowers sway outside
Trapped in my perceived haven
Marooned within my own world
With a cup of St. John's Wort

And a chin left coarsely unshaven.
But I just wished people understood
This syndrome and all the days I felt alone
Because in an under adaptive world
Only knowledge will lead me to a sense of dignity
Allowing me to see little beyond the blanket
And that for the first time in my whole life—
To know what it's like to be free

Daniel North, 2005
Dannorth26@hotmail.co.uk

This poem was taken from the FAAAS (Families of Adults Afflicted with Asperger's Syndrome) Web site (www.faaas.org) and is reproduced with permission from Mr. North.

Dan North wrote "The Blanket" to broaden awareness of AS when the child of a friend was diagnosed as having AS. Its powerful imagery evokes the sense of isolation that is so common in AS. Many adults with AS, even those who marry and have a family, struggle with a sense of being alone and not being understood. And it is not only the person with AS who feels alone. The significant others who live with AS in their midst often feel isolated as well. As the wife of a man with AS put it, "I can never get close to him. It is as if there is a wall of terribly thick glass between us. It makes me feel frustrated, but mostly it makes me lonely and so terribly sad." I believe that the "glass wall" is the result of the lack of understanding between people with AS and people who are NT. We can see one another, but all too often, cannot connect. So many times, when people with AS and NTs interact, both experience the other's behavior as baffling, unpredictable, or even hurtful. It's hard for any of us to connect with people when we can't understand them and often feel hurt by them, so it is not surprising that it is difficult for an NT and a person with AS to connect and feel close. Because of the differences in the way AS and NT brains are structured and the way they function, the two populations experience many situations, especially those involving people, quite differently. The result is what Barbara Jacobs, who wrote *Loving Mr. Spock,* calls "living in parallel universes." When it is not known that AS is playing a role in the relationship, neither the NT nor the person with AS will have a way of knowing about the "parallel universes" and so will assume that the other person's experience is the same as their own. The trouble begins when either the NT or the person with AS behaves according to his understanding of a situation—his "universe." We all make our predictions of other people's behavior based on how we understand the situation and how we ourselves would typically respond to it. Because the universes are different, the behavior will be different and not be what the other person expects. The differences in understanding because of differences in the brains of the AS and the NT means the behavior of either the person with AS or the NT comes as a surprise to the other and is frequently not understood. It may be hurtful as well, particularly since people with AS in many cases cannot predict the impact of their behavior on others. If the NT and the person with AS are in an ongoing relationship, these misunderstandings happen over and over again, and each person becomes less trusting of the other. The relationship becomes more and more damaged. Without a diagnosis, there may be no way to repair the relationship. If the diagnosis is made and acknowledged, it becomes a starting point to explain the difficulties and to hopefully let go of the anger and disappointment both parties usually have. When this happens and if each person begins to understand the "universe" of the other, the differences can be better managed. This result leaves each party free to cherish the relationship and to work together to find solutions to living with AS.

Glossary

Asperger Syndrome (AS): A lifelong neurological condition that causes problems in communications and social interaction and difficulty understanding the minds of others. The condition also tends to results in rigid thinking and, in many cases, an intense focus on a special interest.

Central drive for coherence: The ability to put together different types of information to get a big-picture understanding of a situation. It requires the ability to see the relevance of different types of knowledge to a given problem.

Echolalia: The ability to parrot or mimic someone else's voice, words, speaking pattern, and or mannerisms, often almost perfectly. In autism spectrum disorders (ASD), the individual may recall and perfectly repeat lengthy things they have heard.

fMRI: Functional magnetic resonance imaging is a technology that allows scanning of the brain while it is working. The technology measures neural activity indirectly by detecting associated increases in blood to the areas that are active while the brain is solving problems.

Generalized learning: The ability to take information and skills learned in one situation and apply it to another when needed.

Islets of Ability: The often extraordinary ability of a person with AS to excel in a particular subject while doing much less well in other areas of functioning.

Mind blindness: A term coined by Simon Baron-Cohen, a Cambridge University–based AS researcher, to capture the difficulty those with AS have in understanding that other people have thoughts, feelings, and wishes of their own.

Neurotypical (NT): The designation used to identify those individuals who do not have an autism spectrum disorder.

Nonverbal communication: Information expressed by an individual in a form other than words. It may include the use of gestures, body language, facial expression, and eye contact.

Sensory integration: The process used by the brain to organize sensory input in such a way that the individual can interact with the environment in a meaningful, effective way.

Social echolalia: An adaptive behavior sometimes used by those with AS to manage social situations or, even more broadly, their lives. The behavior consists of studying another person's behaviors, responses, accents, appearance, and interests as a way to manage their own lives.

Special interests: The tendency to become passionately preoccupied in a topic that may be repetitive and quite restrictive. Special interests may focus on almost anything, but frequently involve predictable, controlled, and organized subjects such as trains and rail timetables, etc.

Stim or stimming: A self-stimulating behavior that persons with ASD use to calm themselves in times of stress. When the ASD person is young, it may involve spinning, flapping hands, and rocking. As the person matures, they may discover more socially acceptable repetitive behavior such as rubbing a "lucky stone" or even more complex behaviors such as repetitive computer games.

Theory of mind (TOM): The ability to conceptualize and appreciate the thoughts, wishes, and feelings of another person. The lack of a theory of mind is considered to be a core difficulty in those with AS.

Unconnectivity theory: A theory relating to the possible biological differences in the brain of a person with AS. The theory suggests that the AS brain does not have as extensive connections and as great a capacity for integration of information from various areas of brain function as that of an NT brain.

Resources

Books and Articles

Alvarez A. Reid S. (1999). *Autism and Personality*. London. Routledge.

American Psychiatric Association (2000). *Diagnostic and Statistical Manual of Mental Disorders Text Revision*, 4th ed. (DSM-IV-TR). Washington DC. APA.

Aston M.C. (2000) *The Other Half of Asperger's Syndrome*. London. National Autistic Society.

Aston M.C. (2003) *Asperger's in Love: Couple Relationships and Family Affairs*. London. Jessica Kinglsey Publishers.

Attwood T. (1998) *Asperger's Syndrome: a Guide for Parents and Professionals*. London. Jessica Kingsley Publishers.

Baron-Cohen S. (1995). *Mindblindness—An Essay on Autism and Theory of Mind*. Cambridge. MIT Press.

Baron-Cohen S. (2002). *Mind Reading—The Interactive Guide to Emotions, User Guide and Resource Pack*. Cambridge. University of Cambridge.

Bashe P.R. and Kirby B.L. (2001). *The OASIS Guide to Asperger Syndrome*. New York. Crown Publishers.

Bolick T. (2004) *Aperger Syndrome and Young Children: Building Skills for the Real World*. Gloucester, MA. Fair Winds Press.

Bolick T. (2001) *Asperger Syndrome and Adolescence: Helping Preteens and Teens Get Ready for the Real World*. Gloucester, MA. Fair Winds Press.

California Health and Human Services Agency (1999). *A Report to the Legislature: Changes in the Population of Persons with Autism and Pervasive Development Disorders in California's Developmental Services System: 1987 through 1998.* Sacramento, CA. California Health and Human Services Agency.

Cutler E. (2004). *A Thorn in My Pocket.* Arlington, TX. Future Horizons, Inc.

Damascio A. (1999). *The Feeling of What Happens: Body and Emotion in the Making of Consciousness.* Orlando, FL. Harcourt, Inc.

Fling E. (2000). *Eating an Artichoke.* London. Jessica Kingsley Publishers.

Frith U. (1991). *Autism and Asperger Syndrome.* Cambridge. Cambridge University Press.

Grandin T. (1995). *Thinking in Pictures; and Other Reports from Life with Autism.* New York. Doubleday.

Grandin T. and Johnson C. (2005). *Animals in Translation: Using the Mysteries of Autism to Decode Animal Behavior.* New York. Scribner.

Howlin P. (2004) *Autism and Aperger Syndrome,* second ed. London. Routledge.

Howlin P., Baron-Cohen S. and Hadwin J. (1999). *Teaching Children to Mind-read; A Practical Guide.* Chichester. John Wiley & Sons.

Jacobs B. (2003) *Loving Mr. Spock: the Story of a Different Kind of Love.* London. Penguin Group.

Kanner L. (1973) *Childhood Psychosis: Initial Studies and New Insights.* New York. Winston / Wiley.

Klin A., Volkmar F. R. and Sparrow S. S. (2000) *Asperger's Syndrome*. New York. Guildford Press.

Lawson W. (2003). *Build Your Own Life: A Self Help Guide for Individuals with Asperger's Syndrome*. London: Jessica Kingsley Publishers.

Lawson W. (1998) *Life Behind Glass: A Personal Account of Autistic Spectrum Disorder* Lismore, Australia. Southern Cross University Press.

Myles B.S. and Southwick J. (1999). *Asperger's Syndrome and Difficult Moments: Practical Solutions for Tantrums, Rages, and Meltdowns*. Shawnee Mission, KS. Autism Asperger Publishing Co.

Ratey J.J. (1995). *Neuropsychiatry of Personality Disorders*. Cambridge, MA. Blackwall Science.

Ratey J.J. and Johnson C. (1997). *Shadow Syndromes: The New Forms of Major Mental Disorders that Sabotage Us*. New York: Pantheon Books.

Rodman K. (2003). *Asperger's Syndrome and Adults... Is Anyone Listening? Essays and Poems by Partners, Parents and Family Members of Adults with Asperger's Syndrome*. London. Jessica Kingsley Publishers.

Tatam D. and Prestwood S. (1999) *A Mind of One's Own: A Guide to the Special Difficulties and Needs of the More Able Person with Autism or Asperger's Syndrome,* (3rd ed.) London. The National Autism Society

Willey L. H. (2001) *Asperger's Syndrome in the Family: Redefining the Family.* London. Jessica Kingsley Publishers.

Willey L. H. (1999) *Pretending to be Normal: Living with Asperger's Syndrome.* London. Jessica Kingsley Publishers.

Wing L. and Attwood A. (1987) 'Syndromes of Autism and Atypical Development." In D. Cohen and A. Donnellan, eds., *Handbook of Autism and Pervasive Developmental Disorders.* New York. John Wiley and Sons.

Web sites

ASpar—A support ground and information exchange for people raised by one or more parents with AS: **www.aspar.klattu.com.au**

Asperger Association of New England: **www.aane.org**

Asperger Syndrome Coalition of the United States, Inc. ASC-US: **www.asperger.org**

ASPIRES (Asperger Syndrome Partners and Individuals Resources Encouragement and Support): **www.justgathertogether.com/aspire.html**

Families of Adults Afflicted with Asperger Syndrome: **www.faaas.org**

Liane Holliday Willey's Home Page: **www.aspie.com**

O.A.S.I.S (Online Aspergers Syndrome Information and Support): **www.udel.edu/bkirby/asperger/**

Sensory Integration Resource Center: **www.sinetwork.org**

The Aspen Society of American, Inc. (Asperger Syndrome Education Network): **www.asperger.org**

The Autism Society of America: **www.autism-society.org**

The National Autistic Society: **www.nas.mailbow.ulcc.ac.uk**

Tony Attwood's Home Page: **www.tonyattwood.com**

Yale Child Study Center: **www.autism.fm**

Acknowledgments

I didn't expect to write a book when I first started out on the journey to learn all that I could about AS. When I first heard the term "Asperger's" and read a description of the syndrome, I knew it was something I wanted to understand. I want to thank all the people—patients, professionals, and individuals who live with AS in their lives—for helping me over the years to grasp an understanding of AS.

I'd like to thank Karen Rodman and the Board of Directors of FAAAS for their recommendation of me as a possible author. I'd also like to thank Fair Winds Press, the publisher of this book, and the people there who helped me to make it a reality: Donna Raskin, Wendy Martin (my editor), and John Gettings have all given me support and encouragement.

Three people in particular stand out when I think about my career as a psychologist. These people set the stage for the course of my career: Drs. Leah B. Lapidus, Judith Nowak, and George Nurnberg were all generous teachers who were willing to answer my numerous questions. Warmest thanks to you all.

Thank you, my family and my dear friends. You have always been there for me and believed in me and "my projects," even when it meant some sacrifices for you.

And then there is you, Jake. Our many long talks about our brains and how they work gave me confidence that there are people who are curious about what goes on inside their heads and who might be interested in reading this book. Thanks, Jakester.

About the Author

Juanita P. Lovett, Ph.D., has been a practicing clinical psychologist for twenty-five years. During this time she has worked with clinical groups with an emphasis on adult individuals with Asperger Syndrome (AS) and their spouses/families. She has also taught at the graduate level at both Columbia and Rutgers Universities. She has held appointments on several New Jersey mental health boards, including the Board of the New Jersey Forensic Hospital, and currently serves on the Board of Directors of The Wye River Group on Healthcare and the Foundation for American Health Care Leadership.

Dr. Lovett holds a Ph.D., M. Phil. and M.S. from Columbia University and served a two-year fellowship at The New York Hospital, Cornell—Westchester Division. She is a member of the American Psychological Association, Sigma Xi, and the New York Academy of Science.